CURES &
CURIOSITIES

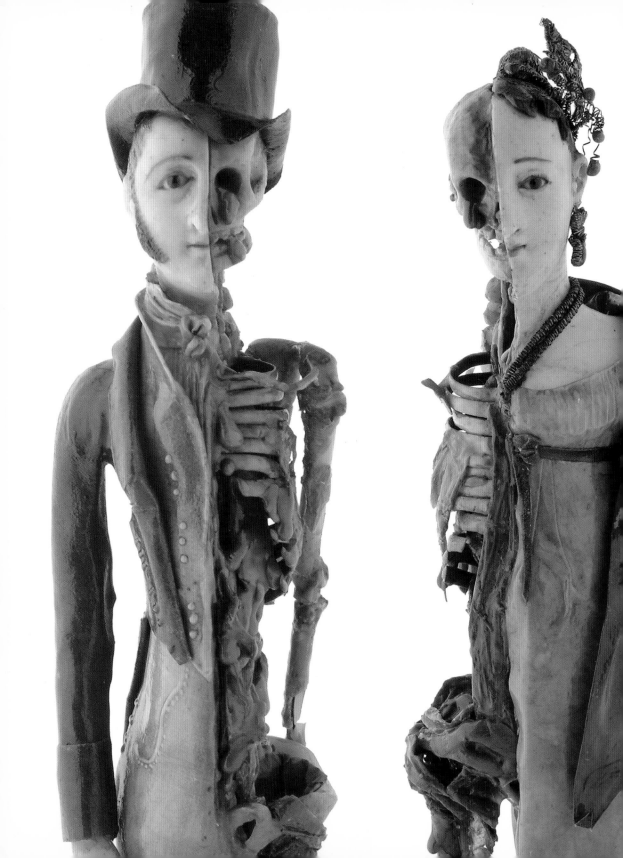

CURES &
CURIOSITIES

INSIDE THE WELLCOME LIBRARY

Compiled & edited by Tony Gould
Foreword by Sebastian Faulks

P

PROFILE BOOKS

First published in Great Britain in 2007 by
Profile Books Ltd
3a Exmouth House
Pine Street
Exmouth Market
London EC1R 0JH
www.profilebooks.com

In association with The Wellcome Trust

The Wellcome Trust is a charity whose mission is to foster
and promote research with the aim of improving human
and animal health.

Wellcome Collection is a new, free, public space devoted
to exploring the links between medicine, life and art.
Three galleries, a range of events and the unrivalled
Wellcome Library root science in the broad context of
health and wellbeing. See www.wellcomecollection.org

10 9 8 7 6 5 4 3 2 1

A CIP catalogue record for this book is available
from the British Library.

ISBN: 978 1 84668 033 5

Editorial consultant: Paul Forty at Brookes Forty
Text and cover design: Rose

Printed and bound in Great Britain by
Butler and Tanner Ltd, Frome and London

CONTENTS

ABOUT THE CONTRIBUTORS

Richard Aspin (Chapter 2, 'Repositories of Domestic Knowledge'; and Chapter 10, 'Doctors at War') is Head of Archives & Manuscripts at the Wellcome Library.

Sarah Bakewell ('Making Honey') is the author of *The Smart: The Story of Margaret Caroline Rudd and the Unfortunate Perreau Brothers* (2001) and *The English Dane: A Life of Jorgen Jorgensen* (2005).

Sebastian Faulks (Foreword) is the author of several novels, including *Birdsong* (1994) and *Human Traces* (2005).

Alice Ford-Smith (Chapter 6, 'Wicked as Ever') is an Assistant Librarian at the Wellcome Library.

Jenny Gould (co-author, with Anne Hardy, of Chapter 5, 'Plagues, Pests and Pollution') has a PhD in history from University College London. Her thesis, on the establishment of the women's military services in Britain, is entitled 'The Women's Corps'.

Tony Gould (Introduction; Chapter 1, 'Collecting the Everyday', co-authored with Ross MacFarlane; and Chapter 15, 'Heat, Dust and Disease') is the author of *A Summer Plague: Polio and Its Survivors* (1995) and *Don't Fence Me In: Leprosy in Modern Times* (2005).

Lesley Hall (Chapter 7, 'Ministering to Minds Diseased'; and Chapter 13, 'Wives, Lovers and Mothers') is a Senior Archivist at the Wellcome Library and author of *Sex, Gender and Social Change in Britain since 1880* (2000) and *Outspoken Women: Women Writing about Sex, 1870–1969* (2005).

Anne Hardy ('Forceful and Forthright: W. H. Bradley'; and co-author with Jenny Gould of Chapter 5, 'Plagues, Pests and Pollution') is Deputy Director of the Wellcome Trust Centre for the History of Medicine at University College, London, and author of *The Epidemic Streets: Infectious Disease and the Rise of Preventive Medicine, 1856–1900* (1993) and *Health and Medicine in Britain since 1860* (2000).

Christopher Hilton (Chapter 8, 'By Land and Sea'; and Chapter 14, 'Hunt the Ancestor') is a Senior Archivist at the Wellcome Library.

Philip Hoare ('The Memory of a Military Hospital') is the author of *Spike Island: The Memory of a Military Hospital* (2002) and *England's Lost Eden: Adventures in a Victorian Utopia* (2005).

Kathryn Hughes ('Mr Beeton's Secret') is the author of *The Short Life and Long Times of Mrs Beeton* (2005).

Douglas Knock (Chapter 11, 'A Quick Fix') is an Assistant Librarian at the Wellcome Library.

Armand Leroi ('The Many Meanings of Monsters') is the author of *Mutants: On the Form, Variety and Errors of the Human Body* (2004) and of the TV Channel 4 documentary series, 'Human Mutants' and 'What Makes Us Human'.

Ross MacFarlane (co-author, with Tony Gould, of Chapter 1, 'Collecting the Everyday') is a Project Archivist/Manager at the Wellcome Library.

Wendy Moore ('News from the Past') is the author of *The Knife Man: Blood, Body-snatching and the Birth of Modern Surgery* (2005).

Robert Olby ('The Roving Intellect of Francis Crick') is the author of *The Path to the Double Helix* (1974/1994) and the *Fontana History of Biology* (2000). He is currently writing a biography of Francis Crick.

Ruth Richardson ('A Serpentine Tale') is the author of *Death, Dissection and the Destitute* (2001).

William Schupbach (Chapter 12, 'Goigs and Thankas') is the Iconographic Collections Librarian at the Wellcome Library and author of *The Paradox of Rembrandt's 'Anatomy of Dr Tulp'* (1982).

Nicolaj Serikoff (Chapter 4, 'A Card Written in Arabic') is the Asian Collections Librarian at the Wellcome Library. He is the editor of *Islamic Calligraphy in the Wellcome Library* (2007).

Julia Sheppard (Chapter 3, 'Breakthroughs and Bust-ups') is Head of Research and Special Collections at the Wellcome Library. She is co-editor of *British Archives: A Guide to Archival Resources in the UK* (4th edition, 2002) and is writing a biography of Silas Mainville Burroughs.

Julianne Simpson (Chapter 9, 'The Elixir of Life') is the Rare Books Librarian at the Wellcome Library.

Gillian Tindall ('Young Doctors in Post-Revolutionary Paris') is the author of *Celestine: voices from a French village* (1994) and *The Journey of Martin Nadaud* (2000) among many other works of non-fiction and fiction.

FOREWORD
by Sebastian Faulks

In the process of researching a novel whose two main characters are Victorian psychiatrists, I spent an evening in 2002 with Dr David Horrobin, a physiologist, writer and entrepreneur. Intimidated by the seemingly boundless extent of his knowledge, I cried out at one point, 'But how do you know all this stuff?' 'Well,' he said, 'the people at the Wellcome Library are awfully helpful.'

A few weeks later, I set out for Euston Road in the company of my general practitioner, Dr Martin Scurr, who had business of his own in the library. It took only a couple of minutes to secure the photo-identity card that let me loose among the stacks, where my first response was one of despair. So compendious was the library's holding on all matters psychiatric that, far from feeling glad that I'd gained free access to an unrivalled resource, I felt only that someone as ignorant as I was had no right to be attempting such a task. I had hardly heard of most of the books; I hadn't read any of them.

At that stage I had perhaps a dozen separate areas of research and I immediately saw that if I was not to be drowned in books I would need to organise my priorities and come again with a more defined reading list. The library's foolproof (believe me) online catalogue did a lot to help me narrow down what I was after.

On my second visit, the panic attack (see under Neurosis and a 'mesh' of related topics) was replaced by something a bit more like a sense of purpose. For a start, the Wellcome looked as a library should, with proper hardwood shelves, the names of great medical figures (Galen, Hippocrates, Fleming) carved into the architrave, and, between the stacks, numerous attractive reading places. Unlike those in the British Library, these seats did not have an exposed and uniform appearance with a sense of bureaucracy looking over one's shoulder for the faintest lapse of protocol – a book returned to the wrong desk or earmarked with the wrong-coloured reservation slip. Nor was it like the London Library, which I love, but which has a choice of tiny schoolboy tables in the labyrinth (I fear if I sit down I may never find my way back) or fat, somniferous armchairs.

The Wellcome offered numerous enticing study possibilities, including small nooks where you could hole up unseen all afternoon and no one would guess you had never had a school lesson in biology. If you needed help in finding or requesting something – and the system did take a little getting used to – the staff would patiently talk you through it or, if you asked nicely and looked suitably hopeless, order it up for you. Uniquely among the libraries I have been to, the Wellcome seemed really to care for the comfort of its readers. One computer terminal was dedicated merely to the remote retrieval of visitors' e-mails, without which the modern student feels that life may be passing him by. The plentiful supply of Wellcome ballpoint pens was another joy, and the tip was just the right width to tackle the crossword in a borrowed moment. The pencils that replaced them are good, as far as pencils go, but not in my view quite the same thing.

So it was that I discovered the joys of opsimathy – a word I think I stumbled on in the library (it means 'learning late in life'). Mornings passed in a small booth watching an entire television series made by Jonathan Miller. A queasy afternoon slipped away as I watched a video of a post-mortem (I had tried to get into a real one, but they are few and hard to find these days). More days than I care to remember dwindled into darkness as I examined brain surgery techniques (Horsley in London, Cushing in America, Wilder Penfield in Montreal) and tried to grasp from ancient learned journals the Victorian view of the inherited element in psychosis and the extent to which Broca's theories of the localization of brain function were accepted. (The Wellcome didn't have a complete run of all the journals, so I went to the library of the Institute of Psychiatry in Denmark Hill, also extremely helpful.)

For those of us who saw three years at university as play-time, the routine and quiet satisfactions of a library day are quite novel. So this, I found myself occasionally thinking, is how my friends passed their student days while I was still in bed. Of course, my student pals would leave their seat every couple of hours and gather in the tea-room to chat or flirt with someone they'd spotted through the stacks, and there was little chance of that at the Wellcome – or not as it was then, anyway. For a cup of tea or sandwich, I had to walk round the oddly refreshment-free streets of north Bloomsbury, where, from one of the foodless thoroughfares, I took the name for the big house in the novel – Torrington, which I turned into a place of plenty. In the end, I usually resorted to Euston station, with its variety of small coffee stalls, though a sandwich from Marks and Spencer's gulped down on the windy forecourt wasn't really what I'd had in mind.

My novel, *Human Traces*, five years in the making, eventually came out in 2005. I could not have written it without the Wellcome Library. I have written another one since, *Engleby* (2007). My foreign rights agent read it and said the person she'd liked most in it was Benny Frost, a minor character in a hospital. I couldn't think who she meant until … Oh yes, Benny – just a walk-on, really. But he owed his life, now I came to think about it, to a footnote in the proceedings of a symposium on personality disorder that I'd read … Where else? In the Wellcome Library.

INTRODUCTION
by Tony Gould

The Wellcome Library is unique. In the field of medical history its only rival in the English-speaking world is the National Library of Medicine in Bethesda, Maryland. But the Wellcome's special collections, in particular, cover a far greater range of material than you would ever expect to find in a medical library. This is due to the vision (or, less flatteringly, acquisitive instincts) of its founder, the pharmaceutical tycoon Henry S. Wellcome, whose mania for collecting is the subject of Chapter 1. The unbelievably rich diversity of manuscripts, books, drawings, paintings and photographs – not to mention the myriad of objects intended for a museum – that Wellcome and his agents gathered from all over Europe, the Middle East, Asia and the Americas ensured that the library which bears his name would never be a narrowly specialist one, as a glance at the chapter headings of this book will attest.

A good library is like an iceberg: the bulk of it is out of sight. Though I have used the Wellcome for a number of years, it was not until I began exploring it for this book that I had any idea of the extent of its collections. As a writer, your research tends to be focused on whatever it is you are writing about (in my case at the Wellcome, it was first polio and then, some years later, leprosy) and you limit your searches to that particular area. So it has been an eye-opener for me to have the freedom to range over any number of subjects and pick and mix, as it were, without fear of being accused of dilettantism.

But the sheer scale of the undertaking was daunting. A friend of mine once unkindly compared a certain Cambridge don writing about Tolstoy to a flea on the back of an elephant, scratching around and saying, 'Hmm, there seems to be a lot of life in here'; and that was rather how I felt as I gazed at the rows of catalogues in the Poynter Room (where studious researchers pore over rare books and barely legible manuscripts under the watchful eye of a curator) and wondered where on earth to begin. My initial excitement soon gave way to despair as I came to realise the immensity of the task I had so blithely taken on. What was I thinking of? How did I ever imagine I could research, let alone write a book that would do anything like justice to the treasure trove that is the Wellcome Library in a matter of six months? Six months? It normally took me years to research and write a book.

Desperate remedies were required. I told Julia Sheppard, the Head of Research and Special Collections whose idea the book was, and who had approached me to do it in the first place, that if it were to be produced in time (for the opening of the Wellcome Collection, as the totally refurbished building that is home to the library was to be called) it could not be done by a single individual; it had to be a team effort.

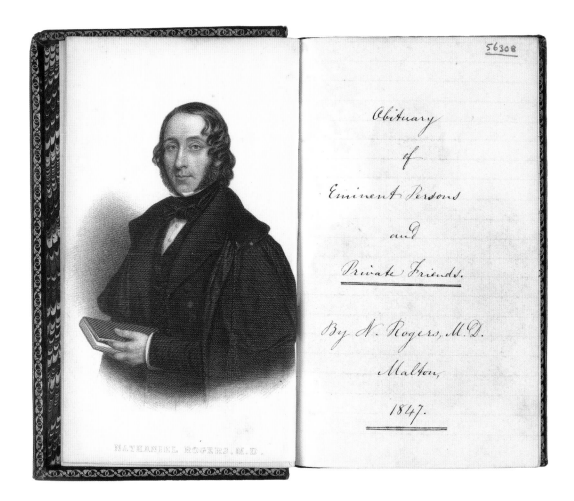

NATHANIEL ROGERS, M.D.

Obituary
of
Eminent Persons
and
Private Friends.

By N. Rogers, M.D.

Malton,

1847.

It was always part of the plan to invite contributions from a few historians and writers who had used the library, but we would also need to draw on the expertise of those librarians and archivists who were most familiar with the collections and ask them to collaborate.

Julia called a meeting and the response was gratifying: almost everyone present volunteered to write, or at least draft, one or more chapters on subjects and themes we discussed, such as war and medicine, travel, alchemy, untimely deaths and executions, sex and birth control, and so on, from the perspective of one or more of the collections in the library. That was the turning point. Despite some further hiccups, from then on it seemed there would be a 'library book' after all, and the closer involvement of library staff in the project was itself a bonus.

At that meeting we considered having a chapter to be called 'Things You Would Not Expect to Find in a Medical Library', but this applied to so many items that have since found their way into existing chapters that eventually we dropped the idea. However, I cannot resist giving a couple of examples here of oddities that would otherwise not be in the book and whose discovery made the random searches of the library's holdings so serendipitous.

The first dates from the middle of the nineteenth century and is entitled 'Obituary of Eminent Persons and Private Friends'.[1] It is compiled by a Dr Nathaniel Rogers and is clearly not his first exercise in the genre. From his current practice in Malton, north Yorkshire, he writes in the preface: 'About twenty years ago, I began to record the deaths of persons distinguished in any of the public walks of life, as well as of members of my own private circle of acquaintance. This volume, still unfinished, is now in London; but after a long interval, I have determined to resume the register with … gratitude to that gracious Providence who, while so many have fallen around, has hitherto preserved the writer.'

The quirkiness of this elegantly bound Volume II, written in an undoctorly neat hand, is in the fortuitous juxtaposition of plumber and duke, of prize-fighter and professor, and in Rogers's own keenness to get in on the act, so to speak. One entry reads in its entirety: 'John S. Rarey, the celebrated horse-farmer, died in America, Oct 4, 1866. I once saw him.' Similarly, of the 4th Duke of Northumberland, he writes: 'During part of the time I spent in Dublin, this nobleman (one of the highest & richest members of the

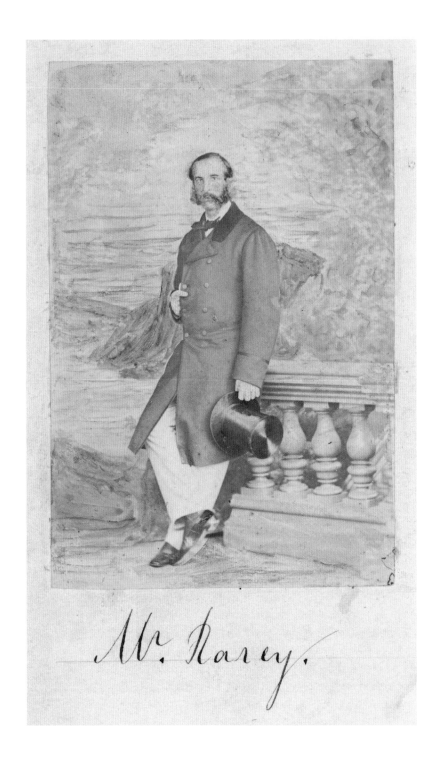

The 'celebrated horse-farmer'
John S. Rarey

peerage) was Lord Lieutenant; and I once saw him, in the Windsor uniform, attending Divine Service with the Duchess, in the Castle Chapel. After an attack of Influenza he was found dead in bed.' But perhaps the most egregious example of squeezing himself into the picture comes in his obituary of a Professor Napier, 'Professor of Conveyancing in the University of Edinburgh; *in which capacity he attached his signature to my diploma'* (my italics).

Yet the book provides fascinating glimpses of nineteenth-century life. David Greenburg, for instance, was a 'coal-porter and prize-fighter of very dissipated habits'. Rogers knew him at Malton 'as a reformed character' and had seen him in the pulpit of the Wesleyan chapel. He goes on: 'Before I left, he married a minister's wife, of some property; but relapsed into habits of intoxication, & died at Scarborough, Dec 28, 1862, aged 47.' Then there is 'Miss Sarah Biffin, who was born without hands or arms, but became a celebrated miniature painter with her toes, [and] died at Liverpool, 2 Oct 1850 aged 66.' Rogers has a good ear. Of Revd John Colliston, minister at Wood Street Chapel, Walthamstow, who died in February 1847, aged 75, he gives the following example of the preacher's 'soft and silken' phraseology: 'Ye must – if you will allow me the expression – ye must be born again!'

Occasionally, Rogers brings to mind Aubrey's *Brief Lives*, as when he writes of one of Napoleon's marshals who died at St Etienne in May 1847 aged 81: 'He was a distinguished officer, but chargeable with indecision; and his non-arrival at the Battle of Waterloo is said to have secured the victory to the English.' He has a nice turn of phrase, too. He says of Mr George Robins, a 'prince of auctioneers' who also died in 1847, leaving his family 'well provided for': 'His advertisements of Property for Sale were drawn up in the language of Romance.' Of what estate agent now could that not serve as an epitaph?

My other example comes from the Royal Army Medical Corps 'Muniment Collection' and is entitled 'The Malingerer's Guide'.[2] Disguised as book matches, hundreds of packets of these guides were air-dropped by the Axis powers among the Allied troops invading Italy in 1944. The soldiers who picked up and opened a box expecting to tear off a match found instead a concertinaed sheet of closely printed instructions on how to fool their medical officers. This elegant piece of propaganda urged the troops to 'come back home alive', cannily pointing out that though the war was nearly over, that only increased the danger, since the death toll was always at its highest towards the end of a war: 'Nobody can say that as a good soldier you haven't done your duty. But no man in the world will ever blame you for not wishing to be one of its last victims … Try the safe turn during these last few weeks, it is far better for you to be a few weeks ill than all your life dead.'

This phrase – 'Better a few weeks ill than all your life dead' – runs through the malingerer's guide like a refrain. Troops are warned not to exaggerate their symptoms, as that will only arouse the medical officer's suspicions. It is important to remember that 'the doctor has the advantage in this game, because he has studied the rules'. So you must: 1) give the impression that you hate to be ill; 2) pick one disease and stick to it; and 3) not tell the doctor too much. This last instruction is crucial; you mustn't know much about the disease you're supposed to be suffering from, and certainly not its name, since doctors don't like you using technical terms: 'You will never be found out if you say too little, but you might easily be caught out if you say too much.'

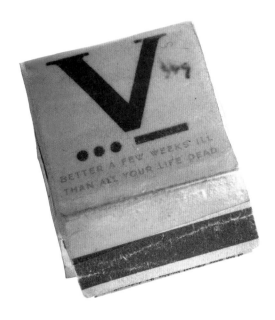

Second World War
Axis propaganda:
'The Malingerer's Guide'
disguised as a book
of matches

The rest of the document is dedicated to specific diseases and how to produce convincing symptoms. If you are faking heart disease, for instance: 'Smoke 20 to 30 cigarettes per day. But if you normally smoke as much, then you might double that number.' (It does not, of course, suggest that if you did that you might really become ill.) Sore throats are not recommended, except for those 'who have still got their tonsils'.

Was 'The Malingerer's Guide' as effective as its ingenuity deserved? Did it increase the number of soldiers reporting on sick parade? Not according to the medical officer who preserved one for posterity. Major A. H. L. Wilson writes that it had 'little or no effect on our troops, though it did enable one man to diagnose, quite correctly, his own disability!'

Cures and Curiosities is a work of celebration. We want to share our delight in the collections and the extraordinary things some of them contain. In the following chapters we explore our chosen themes. These are snapshots; inevitably some areas of the collections are covered better than others; but we never set out to be comprehensive. That is not possible in a book of this kind, which is neither a catalogue nor a guide. Our aim is simply to give the reader a taste of what is available in the Wellcome in the belief that this will act as an incentive for further exploration.

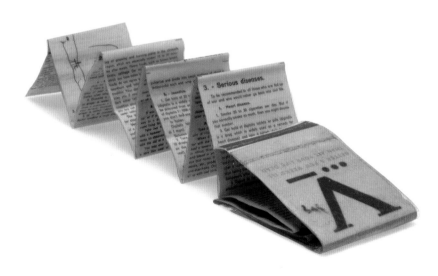

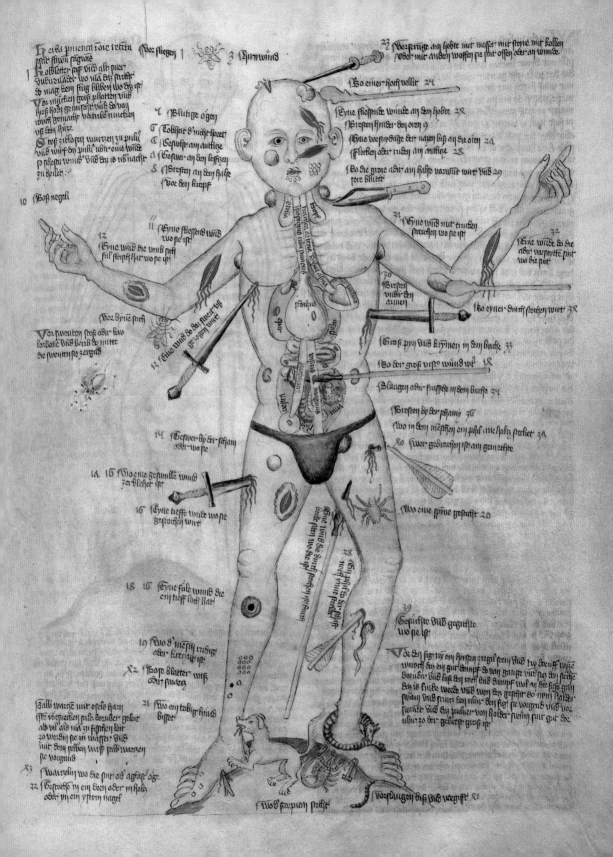

I
COLLECTING
THE EVERYDAY:
HENRY WELLCOME
AND THREE
OF HIS AGENTS

The American-born pharmacist and philanthropist Henry Solomon Wellcome (1853–1936) was always a collector, but it wasn't until after the death in 1895 of his partner in the pharmaceutical firm of Burroughs Wellcome & Co. that he had the freedom and the means to indulge his obsession on an almost industrial scale. By the 1920s he was spending more yearly on acquisitions than the British Museum, and by the early 1930s he had five times as many artefacts as the Louvre. Their value, of course, was by no means comparable. But he was largely indifferent to aesthetic quality and followed the injunction of the nineteenth-century archaeologist and founder of the eponymous Pitt-Rivers museum in Oxford, to 'collect the everyday'.

For a man whose personal papers alone fill nearly 700 archive boxes and require four volumes, amounting to 728 pages, to catalogue some 6,500 separate items, Henry Wellcome remains a remarkably elusive figure.[1] There is something Gatsby-like in this, as in his humble mid-western origins and propensity for giving large parties attended by everybody who was anybody. But there the resemblance most decidedly ends. Wellcome belongs to an earlier, sturdier generation than F. Scott Fitzgerald's protagonist and his romantic idealism was underpinned by hard-headed and shrewd business acumen.

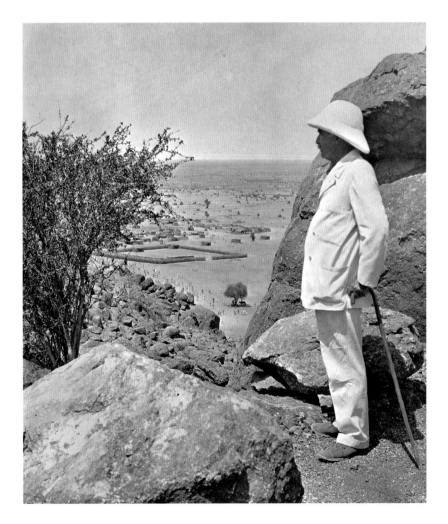

Previous page:
Wound-man, with multiple injuries, from one of Henry Wellcome's early acquisitions, a mediaeval German 'Apocalypse' (c. 1420–30)

Left:
Wellcome overseeing excavations at the archaeological site he financed at Jebel Moya in the Sudan, 1913–14

While his public life as a captain of industry was rich, various and successful (though honours came late to this long-naturalised British citizen), his private life was marked by failure and disappointment. His friendship with his fellow American émigré, Silas Burroughs, turned sourly litigious and threatened their business partnership well before the latter's fortuitously early death. His marriage to the philanthropist Dr Barnardo's daughter Syrie, who was less than half his age at the time, ended in separation and, later, divorce when Syrie had a daughter with Somerset Maugham (whom she then married and whose name she would bear for the rest of her life though they, too, separated). Wellcome got custody of their only child, a son he'd named Henry Mounteney after his friends the explorers Henry Morton Stanley and Mounteney Jephson, but in him, too, he was to be disappointed. The boy Mounteney suffered from what would now probably be diagnosed as dyslexia, but what was then labelled 'backwardness'. This meant that he could never be the heir that Wellcome had wanted, though he would lead a contented life as a farmer and family man.

My plans exist in my mind like
a jig-saw puzzle, and gradually
I shall be able to piece it together.

Henry Wellcome, as recalled by his deputy and general manager,
George Pearson, 12 December 1940

Collecting 'curios'

Though he never became a recluse, the once outgoing and gregarious American from a poor home in the mid-west grew ever more inward-looking and isolated as a result of his bitter personal experiences. Increasingly, he sought solace in work, philanthropy and travel – which for him was simply another kind of work. As Syrie would complain to an intermediary after Wellcome, suspecting her of the ultimate crime (in his eyes) of infidelity, had dumped her, 'ever since our marriage, the greater part of our time had been spent

… in places I *detested*, collecting curios.' Given that the attraction of collecting for him was more in the acquisition of objects rather than in what became of them – at his death thousands of unopened boxes were found stored away in piles – the spirited Syrie could be forgiven for suspecting that for him she herself might be little more than one of his 'curios'.

Henry Wellcome was curiously lonely …
It may be doubted whether anyone knew
him with sufficient intimacy to do more
than speculate as to his real feelings
and motives.

Sir Henry Dale, obituary in *The Times*, 1 August 1936

In the early days at least, Wellcome's journeys to Nice, Biarritz, Vienna and all the other places that Syrie claimed to detest gave him the freedom that he didn't have in London to pursue his collecting mania incognito. At home he tried to preserve his anonymity by acting through agents. If he visited the book stalls himself, he told an American friend, 'I usually put on very plain clothes … A top hat usually excites the cupidity of the dealer, and the higher the hat the higher the price.' But once his Historical Medical Museum became a reality (even if it was not open to the public), dealers got wise to his methods and could usually spot his agents. Many are the tales of young and innocent members of staff sworn to secrecy setting out on their first cloak-and-dagger mission only to discover that the dealers were well aware of their identity and sometimes even phoned confirmation to the Wellcome without bothering to inform them first!

One of the things about Sir Henry
was that he thought he would never die.

W. J. Britchford, an employee for 44 years, in a letter dated 29 April 1975

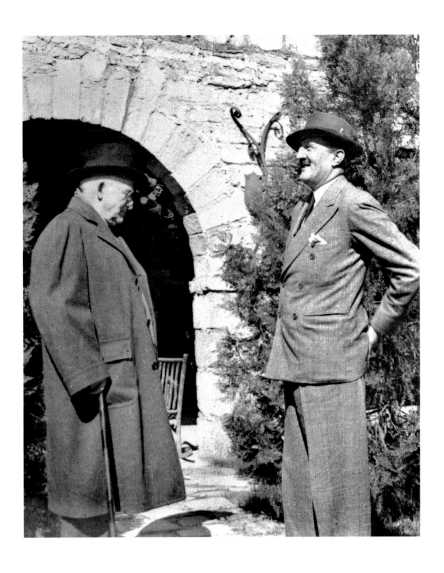

Sir Henry Wellcome (left), shortly before his death in 1936, with his 'Foreign Secretary', Peter Johnston-Saint

Wellcome traced his interest in collecting back to the occasion in his early childhood when his father showed him a 'relic' in the shape of a sharpened flint. His first contact with American Indians was a hostile one, when as an eight-year-old in Garden City, Minnesota, he helped his doctor uncle treat people wounded in the Sioux uprising of 1862. This made an indelible impression on him, but his early hatred of Native Americans soon turned to respect and sympathy for their plight, which – being Wellcome – he expressed philanthropically, giving long-term financial and other forms of aid to the lay missionary William Duncan (1832–1918) and his Metlakahtla settlement in British Columbia and then in Alaska.[2] His anthropological approach to history may well have stemmed from this early exposure to so-called 'primitive' people.

He had started as a genuine collector, but it had become a magpie collection. He could not leave anything alone in his field. He lost the medical and historical science theme and would collect anything. He was a cosmopolitan collector. He had no business to be collecting armour and judging by the sales, it was rather bad European armour. I don't know why he ever acquired certain good collections, for example prehistoric axes, except for the fact that he had advice from a man on the staff who was an expert on prehistoric matters.

L. G. Matthews, a Director of the Wellcome Foundation from 1944 to 1960
(A. D. Lacaille was archaeologist at the Wellcome Museum from 1928 to 1959)

It wasn't until he had the idea of holding a historical medical exhibition to celebrate the first quarter century of Burroughs Wellcome & Co.'s existence that Wellcome began seriously to specialise in medical history. Even then he interpreted the subject so broadly that it encompassed an ever-widening array of allied subjects.

As more and more material poured in, the Historical Medical Exhibition developed into a Historical Medical Museum, a small part of which was given over to books and manuscripts. But he was thwarted in his ultimate ambition to create a Museum of Man. After his death his trustees spent years rationalising his mammoth collection of disparate artefacts, offloading whole segments that were devoted to arms and armour and the like to other museums and, finally, even the medical material, most of which is now on permanent loan to the Science Museum. Given Wellcome's own priorities, it is a touch ironic that the lasting memorial of his passion for collecting should be a library rather than a museum. Nonetheless the Wellcome Library remains very much his creation, its broad interpretation of what constitutes medical history owing everything to his initial vision – and surpassing wealth.

He always managed to convey his vision of 'great things' in the future to his staff, and I think others shared my own view that it was this alone which kept us with him, for the appalling working conditions, the irritation and embarrassments of the anonymity and pseudo-secrecy which was enforced even in our personal relations with professional colleagues in other institutions, together with the apparently unending task of sorting vast and ever-growing quantities of materials, often made our loyalty seem misguided. Wellcome was one of those who find the journey more interesting than the end, and he found collecting more satisfying than the task of organising the collection into a well-planned museum.

Noel Poynter, Director of the Museum and Library, Report to the Trustees, 6 February 1964

The Curator:
C. J. S. Thompson (1862–1943)

The son of a pharmacist in Liverpool, Charles Thompson followed in his father's footsteps and qualified as a chemist and druggist, but he never practised, preferring to pursue the career of a pharmaceutical writer and journalist. A series of practical handbooks that he produced in the 1890s caught Henry Wellcome's eye and led to his employment in a rather nebulous capacity 'in connection with literary and other work'. In effect, his appointment at the turn of the century marks Wellcome's transition from amateur to professional collector, and Thompson became his new employer's principal agent. His earliest recorded acquisition for Wellcome was made in 1897.

In addition to his collecting activities, Thompson wrote a number of historical medical booklets for Burroughs Wellcome & Co. to distribute at medical congresses. These were anonymous, but at the same time he was publishing romantic novels under a variety of pseudonyms – presumably to prevent Wellcome, who frowned on any moonlighting by his employees, from finding out. His extramural writing, when it did finally come to Wellcome's notice, ruptured their relations and put an end to his employment; but that was not until 1925, by which time he had worked for Wellcome for a quarter of a century and been curator of his Historical Medical Museum for all fourteen years of its existence.

A penchant for pseudonyms would have appealed to the secretive Wellcome when it came to collecting, and Thompson was adept at coming up with them. The Munich book dealer M. L. Ettinghausen found himself doing so much business with the firm of Epworth & Co. that he decided to visit their offices when he was in London. He made his way to Newman Street and was surprised to find that they consisted of a single locked room on the second floor of a building. The caretaker told him the owner only ever came to collect his letters and parcels. Ettinghausen looked through the letter box and saw 'nothing but bare walls', as he wrote in his memoirs. 'The firm remained most mysterious, till one day some book was returned by them and I found the paper used for packing came from Burroughs Wellcome & Co.' Epworth was Thompson's elder brother's first name.

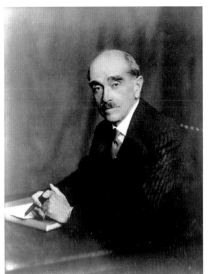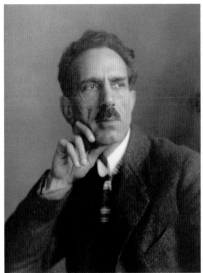

Though he was pensioned off and cold-shouldered by Wellcome, Thompson did not go into a decline. He became honorary curator of the historical collections of the Royal College of Surgeons and continued to produce popular books until his death. His wife of fifty years outlived him and the film director Paul Rotha was one of his four children.

The Orientalist: Dr Paira Mall (1874–1957)

The Wellcome's extensive and valuable collection of Asian manuscripts, books and images is built on the foundations laid by a man who, even before he joined Wellcome's staff in 1910, had had 'a rather remarkable career', as C. J. S. Thompson informed his boss. Of 'Hindoo extraction', Paira Mall had been brought up by an English lady who wanted him to be a missionary. But he had other ideas. He studied medicine in Munich and found his way back to India, where he became medical adviser to the Maharajah of Kapurthala. He took time off to serve as a surgeon in the Japanese army during the Russo-Japanese war of 1904–05 before returning to Kapurthala and thence to England, where his medical training, outstanding linguistic ability and familiarity with Indian palaces and temples strongly recommended him to Wellcome, who promptly sent him back to India as his collecting agent there.

Paira Mall did not have a free hand, though. Before purchasing any item costing £3 or more he had to cable London for approval, which – in the early days at least – was not always forthcoming. On 21 June 1911 Thompson wrote to him sternly: 'With respect to the prolongation of your journey Mr Wellcome wishes to see further the result of your work before coming to a decision … He desires me to point out to you that of course the expense of the journey is very great, and he naturally expects an adequate return for the outlay. I am sorry to say that so far he is disappointed with the result, and if a better return is not likely to follow later on, he might find it necessary to recall you.' Apparently Mall had been sending home too many 'charms' of 'the lingam and phallic type'.[3]

Yet he must have been doing something right, for he remained in Wellcome's employment for sixteen years, no fewer than ten of which were spent travelling the length and breadth of the subcontinent, collecting objects and artefacts as well as manuscripts and books and visiting such remote Himalayan fastnesses as Nepal and Ladakh, where he was able to acquire rare and valuable manuscripts, as well as such bizarre objects as a Tibetan lama's drum made out of a child's cranium.

Though he was finally recalled at the end of the First World War, Mall did not arrive in England until 1921 – it took him that long to gather and transport the plethora of material he had collected to Bombay for shipping to London. His job was done, but his vast collection would not be fully catalogued in his lifetime. 'Indeed,' the former curator of the Wellcome Library Oriental Collections, Nigel Allan, recalls in *Pearls of the Orient: Asian Treasure from the Wellcome Library* (2003), 'many cases of oriental manuscripts remained in the newspapers in which they had been wrapped during the early part of the century until the 1970s.'

The Foreign Secretary:
Captain Peter Johnston-Saint (1886–1974)

Saint, as he is sometimes referred to, had qualities in common with his fictional namesake, Leslie Charteris's 'The Saint'. Ex-Indian Army and Royal Flying Corps, he was handsome, dashing, with a love of sports cars, and well-connected – Queen Victoria's granddaughter, Princess Ena of Battenberg, was a childhood acquaintance 'at Balmoral' who later became Queen of Spain and proved a useful contact when Johnston-Saint was casting a covetous eye on the superannuated historical artefacts of the Royal Pharmacy in Madrid in 1928. And at a dinner party in Delhi in 1934 we find him hobnobbing – if only briefly – with the Viceroy of India, Lord Willingdon.

My chief difficulty in associating with medical men or officers in this country [India] has been to dissociate the work which we are doing from the trade or business aspect.

For instance, in conversation with the Chief of the Army Medical Staff to-day, he said to me, 'Oh, yes, I know your preparations well, they are excellent.'

And another medico said, 'Your representative calls to see me from time to time.'

They don't seem to understand that the WRI [Wellcome Research Institution] is quite a separate affair and all seem to have the idea that it is a branch of the business of Burroughs Wellcome & Co. ...

Peter Johnston-Saint's diary, Delhi, India, 10 February 1934

The Queen [of Spain] told me that even to-day a concoction of Orange water or Lemon water was largely used in Spain as a nerve sedative and recalled to me that when the bomb was thrown at her on her wedding day, the first thing she was given was some of this Orange water.

Peter Johnston-Saint's diary, Audience with the Queen, Madrid, 6 February 1928

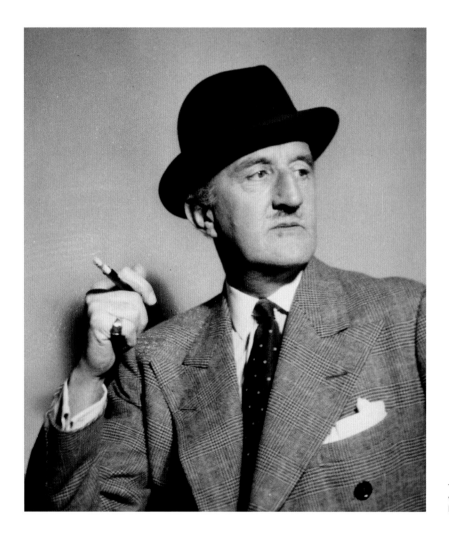

The dashing and well-connected Captain Peter Johnston-Saint

In searching the old town [of Tarbes] I came across a curious old shop where they sold spectacles, kept by an old woman. The shop had one window and without exaggeration one might say that the things therein had not been changed or dusted or cleaned for at least 25 years. The door bore a porcelain plate saying that the Maison was founded in 1825. I went in and grubbing amongst the things there I found a curious old pair of spectacles and two very old pairs of pince nez, also a curious leather appliance for placing over the eyes after an operation. I bought the lot for Fr 25 (4/2d). As it was late now I returned home.

Peter Johnston-Saint's diary, Spectacles, Tarbes, SW France, 21 March 1928

Johnston-Saint joined the Wellcome Research Institution in 1921 and became Thompson's second-in-command at the museum. His work in assembling material for the Joseph Lister centenary exhibition, combined no doubt with his social graces, led to his promotion to 'Foreign Secretary', a post that enabled him to devote all his time to travelling and collecting for the museum, at first in Europe and then further afield. His diaries are full of interesting observations; they have been described as 'a minor classic of inter-war travel literature' and in the 1940s he did publish two travel books, *Green Hills and Golden Sands* and *Castanets and Carnations*.[4]

His work in gathering the memorabilia of French medical men, including the Dr Gachet who treated Van Gogh for self-inflicted wounds and became his friend – and the subject of Van Gogh's sole etching, a print of which Johnston-Saint purchased for under £6[5] – so impressed the French government that they appointed both him

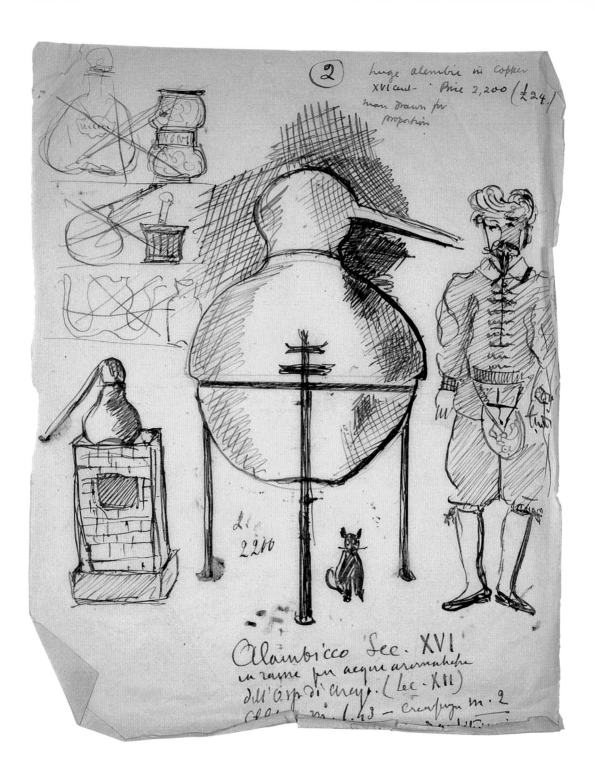

and Henry Wellcome to the Légion d'Honneur. But after Wellcome's death, Johnston-Saint found himself in the awkward position of dismantler-in-chief of collections of objects that, even if he had not been instrumental in gathering them in the first place, had formed part of his respected employer's master plan. The gradual but inexorable depletion of the museum and its staff eventually wore him down and, in the words of the librarian John Symons, he 'retired in bitter disappointment'.

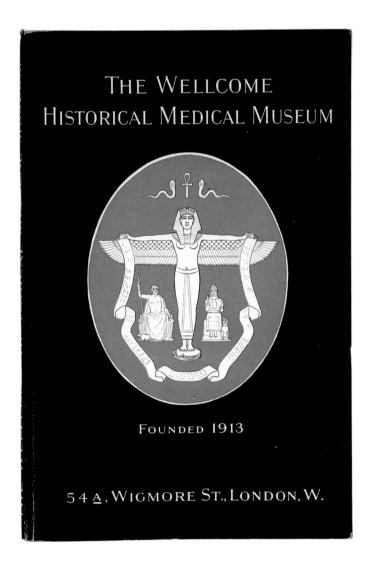

Left:
Johnston-Saint's sketches of objects offered to him for sale in Rome

Right:
The front cover of the handbook to The Wellcome Historical Medical Museum, 1920

THE WELLCOME HISTORICAL MEDICAL MUSEUM

FOUNDED 1913

54 A. WIGMORE ST., LONDON, W.

A Medecine to cure a face that is Redd, and full of Pimples ~ ~ ~

Take two penny worthe of Quicksiluer, putt it in a litle glasse add thereto so much fasting Spitle as will serue to kill it, then shake them well togeather, and the quicksiluer when it is killed will looke like auste: Then take such a Stone as Paynters do grynde theire coulors vppon, beyng cleane washed, and take of the Oyle of Bayes the quantity of a good Aple, Grinde your Quicksyluer and it togeather vppon the Stone, and temper it still with woodbynde water and so grynde it vntill the Oyntement do looke very graye then putt it in a Boxe, and annoynte your face therewith euery euening and morning for the space of 14 dayes keeping your selfe close in your chamber all that tyme, and vsing the drinck following one weeke before you applye the Oyntement, all the tyme you do apply it, and one weeke after viz Take a quantity of new Brane and to euery tenn gallons take halfe a pounde of Madder, stirr these well togeather, and putt them in a vessell and when it is stale drinck thereof both morning and euoning and diuers tymes in the daye. These beyng vsed as is aforesaid will by Gods helpe heale it. But for a Seuennighte your face will Looke worse then before, vntill such tyme as the humor be killed, that is betwixte the fleshe and the skinn. ~

2
REPOSITORIES OF DOMESTIC KNOWLEDGE: THE EVOLUTION OF RECIPE AND REMEDY BOOKS

Recipes are at the heart of the Wellcome Library's collections. The oldest European artefact in the library is a parchment list of Old English folk remedies from about 1000 AD.[1] The earliest documented library acquisition by Henry Wellcome was the recipe book of Lady Ayscough in 1897.[2] Compiling and collecting recipes for medical complaints or for the kitchen is the very essence of healthcare and maintaining wellbeing down the centuries. Small wonder then that the Wellcome Library holds an unrivalled collection of medical and culinary recipes, in mediaeval leechbooks, household and family compilations from the sixteenth to the nineteenth centuries, and printed works from the fifteenth century onwards.

M anuscript recipe books began to be acquired by Henry Wellcome and his agents from several sources, including London salerooms, book dealers and private treaty sales, at the very end of the nineteenth century. Originally they would have formed part of a larger assemblage of family papers, but most of them had already been removed from their context by the time they were acquired. So they came to the Wellcome as single items, and many are difficult now to identify with known families or even to localise in a particular part of the country.

At the time of Wellcome's death in 1936 there were probably between 150 and 200 such books in the collection, depending on how they are defined. Thirty or so of these came from the cookery book collection of John Hodgkin of Reading (1857–1930), purchased at Hodgson's auctioneers in London in April 1931. Collecting activity fell away after 1936 across the library, and when it began again in earnest in the 1950s the focus was predominantly on professional and establishment medicine. Not more than a dozen English manuscript recipe books appear to have been acquired between 1936 and 1986. There was no evident scholarly interest in the history of domestic medicine, and it was not even clear that cookery was a relevant subject for a medical library.

The growth of the collection during the past two decades, during which some eighty additional manuscripts have been acquired, was fuelled by changing patterns of historical research, the altered status of orthodox medicine and its alternatives, and the recent development of new outreach and access priorities in research libraries. From the 1990s academic historians have increasingly turned their attention to manuscript recipe collections to illuminate everyday life in pre-industrial England and to investigate the role of laymen and women in delivering early modern healthcare.

This development encouraged the library to acquire more recipe books, whilst at the same time increasing the visibility of the collection and stimulating the interest of a wider circle of potential users – herbalists, cookery writers, amateur historians of all sorts. Medicine, which used to be the preserve of the various medical professions, has become more democratic, and consequently the historical record of lay medical activity seems more relevant and absorbing to current historians, practitioners and patients, actual

Previous page:
A page from Ann Dacre's book, 1606

Opposite:
A page from Lady Ayscough's 'Receits of phisick and chirurgery', 1692, Henry Wellcome's earliest documented library acquisition

Mr John Wooddalls receit to cure all Itchings in the Eyes smartings immoderate rheumes and Ophathalmies at ye begining wch doth well strengthen ye Sight

R: Vitreolum album pulverisate ʒ1; one new laid Egge boyle ye Egge hard, shell it and cleave it through; take out ye Yolk and in place thereof put ye Copperus powdered; let it soe remaine closed 2 houres or more, then put it into a cleane soft ragge being still soe closed together and straine it hard; and water will come forth of a greene colour, keep it in a glass close stopped, and when Occasion is drop a drop or 2 into your Eyes

---

For a wheizing in ye Pipes or Lungs

R: Raisins of ye Sunn stone and stamp them and take their Weight in double refined Sugar and incorporate them to a Conserve and take ye Quantity of a beane morning and evening and stroke downe ye Stomack every morning constantly

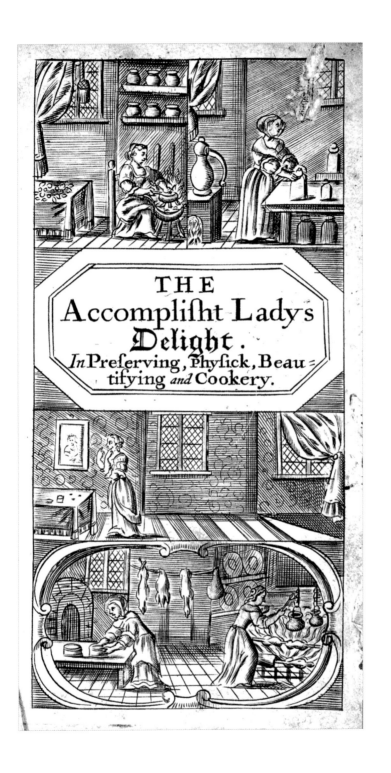

THE
Accomplisht Lady's
Delight.
In Preserving, Physick, Beau=
tifying *and* Cookery.

The title page of
'The Accomplisht Ladys
Delight', 1675, attributed to
Hannah Wolley, an example
of the early printed books
that gradually replaced
manuscript books

or potential. And though early modern recipes are not always intelligible, they are usually in English and often replete with a winning combination of earthy language and bizarre or disgusting ingredients. It is not difficult to justify the continued acquisition of a genre of manuscript that is now the most heavily used in the Wellcome Library. There are still many such manuscripts in private hands and they appear regularly in salerooms and via dealers. The collection will continue to grow in future years.

> *A medicine for a quinzey or swellinge*
> *of the Kernelles in the throwte.*
> *Take a redd Cock of an yeare olde or more,*
> *cutt of the legges and Slytt hym in the Back,*
> *and so lay hym about the sorre part of your*
> *neck, the guttes and all as warme as you can,*
> *and lett it lye there for the space of 12 howers*
> *and it will asswage your kernelles.*
>
> From Anne Dacre's book, 1606

A noble or genteel practice

Although lay recipe collections survive from the sixteenth century, the practice of recording medicinal and culinary recipes in England seems to have been a seventeenth-century development. At first it is particularly associated with noble or genteel households, sometimes Roman Catholic or at least High Anglican. Indeed the earliest compilation in the Wellcome Library, dated 1606, is the recipe collection of Anne Dacre (1557–1630), Countess of Arundel, widow of Philip Howard (1557–1595), 1st Earl of Arundel and Surrey.[3] Anne Dacre was a noted lay medical practitioner and herbalist, who ministered to a large number of supplicants, and compounded and dispensed drugs. Some of her recipes remained in currency throughout the seventeenth century, and are found ascribed to her in both manuscript and printed compilations. She was also a Roman Catholic convert and priest harbourer, and confidante of Mary Queen of Scots.

Other seventeenth-century compilations in the collection associated with the well-born include Lady Frances Catchmay's book, c. 1625,[4] the volumes belonging to Philip Stanhope (1584–1656), 1st Earl of Chesterfield, compiled c. 1635,[5] the book owned by Rhoda Hussey (d. 1686), wife of Lord Ferdinando Fairfax of Cameron (1584–1648),[6] the recipe book of Katherine Jones (1614–91), Lady Ranelagh, sister of Robert Boyle,[7] and the compilation ascribed to Joanna St John, c. 1680, daughter of Sir Oliver St John (1598–1673), Lord Chief Justice.[8]

In keeping with the elevated social standing of some of the earlier compilers and owners of recipe books, recipes could be acquired not only from the immediate family circle and community, but from far afield, even overseas. Sarah Hughes's book, dated 1637, includes a section in Spanish headed *libro de recetas de Portugal para hacer peuetas y pastillas y adreçar guantes perfumados* – 'a recipe book from Portugal for making scented sticks and cakes and preparing perfumed gloves'.[9] Ann Fanshawe (1625–80), whose husband Sir Richard Fanshawe (1608–66) served as Charles II's ambassador at Madrid and Lisbon in the 1660s, included several Spanish culinary recipes in her book, among them chocolate and what has been claimed to be the earliest English recipe for ice cream.[10]

But the recipe book of Margaret Paston, eldest daughter of Robert Paston (1631–83), 1st Earl of Yarmouth, shows evidence of trade in the opposite direction.[11] Margaret married a Venetian nobleman, Girolamo Alberto di Conti, and her book, transcribed into Italian in the 1680s, apparently in her own hand, contains numerous references to Paston family recipes and other English sources, and was perhaps written for Margaret's Italian household and adopted family. She had had some contact before marriage with members of the Royal Society, and seems to have compounded medicines in her own laboratory.

A page from Lady Ann Fanshawe's recipe book, c.1664, with a sketch of a chocolate pot

To make Almon Milk called
Garapiña de Leche de Amendas

Madrid 10
Augt 1665

Boyle 5 qts of yᵉ best fountaine water, wᵗʰ a quarter
of an ounce of whole sinamon in it, a quarter
of an houre then poure it into an Earthen
pan in wᶜʰ there is 3 pounds of Almonds
beat small, after hauing them been blanched
& beat wᵗʰ Orange flowre water, stirr them
well together & lett them stand 2 houres, &
put into it a pound of yᵉ best white sugar
well beat, then strane it through (a thick
Canvas stramer & put in a draghme of
. . . . . Greece, if you like it, put it into a
. . . . . . ottle. & sett it in a Coole sellar
. . . . . . e it after 4 houres standing
. . . . . . keep good 2 days, & 2 nights
. . . . . . r.

To dresse Chocolatte. 23

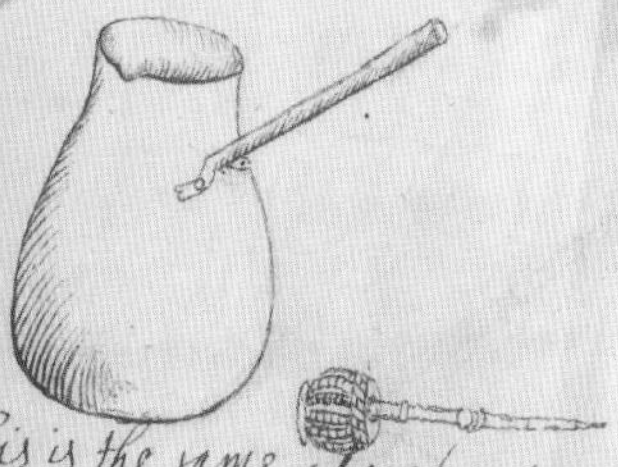

this is the same
that are mayd in the
Indis

chocolay pots

[remaining lines illegible shorthand]

As the seventeenth century progresses, the number of surviving manuscript recipe books increases, and the social range of compilers and owners widens. Rising population, prosperity and literacy during the century would be enough to account for the increase in quantity, but the widening social span may also have had something to do with the middling sort aping the habits of their betters. Certainly recipes seem to have been especially prized if they could be ascribed to a noble or otherwise high status source or authority, as they often were – 'sent to my sister Cartwright by her neece the Duchess of Buckingham'.

To make Icy Cream.
Take three pints of the best cream, boyle it with a blade of Mace, or else perfume it with orang flowerwater or Ambergreece, sweeten the cream with sugar, let it stand till it is quite cold, then put it into Boxes, either of Silver or tinn, then take Ice chopped into small peeces and putt it into a tub and set the Boxes in the ice covering them all over, and let them stand in the Ice two hours, and the Cream Will come to be Ice in the Boxes, then turne them out into a salver with some of the same Seasoned Cream, so serve it up at the Table.

From Ann Fanshawe's book, c. 1664

A currency of exchange

Recipes, both medicinal and culinary, were a currency of exchange within and between families and other social networks, and their circulation oiled the wheels of friendship, cemented generational ties and marked the union of families. Lady Catchmay's book was one of several she owned that she instructed her son to have copied and distributed to her other offspring. Ann Fanshawe's book seems to have been conceived as a recapitulation of domestic knowledge, much of which derived from Ann's own mother, written out by a professional scribe for the benefit of her own children (it was ultimately inherited by her daughter Katherine, as recorded in her ownership inscription). Anne Dacre's recipe book is dated the same year that her son married Alathea Talbot (d.1654) and was evidently produced as a wedding gift for her new daughter-in law. Katharine Palmer's book is dated 1700, the year she married Ralph Palmer (1678–1755), great-nephew of Baldwin Hamey (1600–1676) the younger.[12]

Early modern recipe compilations are therefore much more than mere practical manuals. Indeed, it might be doubted how far they are practical tools at all, with the remedies almost invariably lacking formula, directive and dosage, and the culinary recipes precise quantities of ingredients and directions for cooking. They are primarily repositories of domestic knowledge, household practice and family association, contributed to by both women and men, whose chief function was to serve as a record of use, transmission and exchange of recipes. How else to explain the frequency with which they were copied, redacted, gifted and bequeathed, or the importance assigned to the sources of recipes?

Elizabeth Okeover, who contributed to her family repository in the late seventeenth century, ascribed recipes variously to 'Aunt E:O', 'Aunt L:O', to a 'Coz: Okeover', to her father and mother, and to an 'Unkle Rudyerd'.[13] Another contributor had so little interest in the meaning of the recipes she transcribed from another Okeover family book in the collection that she missed out two entire pages of text without apparently noticing. Though recipes were tried out and used, as we know from the frequent annotations in recipe books as to their efficacy or otherwise – 'this one I make', '… hath often been experienced by my Cozin …', etc. – and the crossing out of failed recipes, the recipe book does not seem to have been the manual that would have been to hand at the kitchen hearth or in the stillroom. Practical, how-to-do-it knowledge depended on skills imparted orally and demonstrably.

A Restorative Snail Water.
Take a peck of garden snails, wash them in
4 or 5 waters afterwards in small beer pound
them shells and all then take a quart of earth
worms and scower them with salt and chop
them in peices then take angelica Egremony
sallendine red burdock roots rosemary wood
sorrell ye inner rind of a barberry tree of each
a handfull rue and baresfoot of each half
a handfull 2 drams of saffron 5 ounces of
Hartshorne fenegrid and turmerick of each
one ounce and 2 grams of Cloves. Steep all
in a earthen vessell close stopt 24 hours in two
gallons of strong beer and a gallon and half of
strong white wine and then distill in a worme
or an alembeck remember before you distill
it to steep your saffron over night in a quart
of your white wine.

From Eliz. Smith's book, 1700[14]

RECIPE RELATED COLLECTIONS

Despite the vigour of the manuscript culture of early modern England, in which medicinal and culinary recipes formed a significant part of the popular medium of exchange, the period was of course one of increasing printed book production. Manuscript recipe books have their counterpart in print, and the two are often closely interlinked, recipes being borrowed and traded back and forth, with or without attribution. The Wellcome Library has a fine collection of English printed recipe and household books from the sixteenth to the nineteenth century, which complement and contextualise the manuscripts.

Printed recipe books

The earliest printed works of this genre were authored by men though often explicitly directed at a female readership, for example Sir Hugh Platt's *Delightes for Ladies, to adorne their Persons, Tables, Closets, and Distillatories* (1611). Later in the seventeenth century female authorship became acceptable, at first in the form of indirect attribution, as in Elizabeth Countess of Kent's *A choice Manual or rare and select Secrets in Physick and Chirurgery* (1653), the first medical book printed in England attributed to a named woman, albeit posthumously. Later still, female authorship was more explicit, as in Hannah Wolley's several works (published from 1661 onwards) or Mary Kettilby's *A collection of above three hundred receipts in cookery, physick, and surgery* (1714).

The evolution of printed recipe books over the early modern period more closely mirrors the changing patterns of medical politics and gender relations than do manuscript compilations. Printed works are *ipso facto* public claims to knowledge and expertise and statements of opinion that provide opportunities for advertising political and other positions, but also carry risks of public censure.

At first printed recipe books were typically attributed to noblewomen or households, and often assumed a high-class readership. As the anonymous editor of *The Queens Closet Opened* (1654) wrote in his preface, 'what can be more noble than that which

THE

PROFESSED COOK:

OR, THE MODERN ART OF

Cookery, Paſtry, and Confectionary,

MADE PLAIN AND EASY.

Conſiſting of the moſt approved Methods in the

FRENCH as well as ENGLISH COOKERY.

IN WHICH

The French Names of all the different Diſhes are given and explained,
whereby every Bill of Fare becomes intelligible and familiar.

CONTAINING

I. Of Soups, Gravy, Cullis and Broths.
II. Of Sauces.
III. The different Ways of dreſſing Beef,
   Veal, Mutton, Pork, Lamb, &c.
IV. Of Firſt Courſe Diſhes.
V. Of dreſſing Poultry.
VI. Of Veniſon.
VII. Of Game of all Sorts.
VIII. Of Ragouts, Collops, and Fries.
IX. Of dreſſing all Kinds of Fiſh.
X. Of Paſtry of different Kinds.
XI. Of Entremets, or laſt Courſe Diſhes.
XII. Of Omelets.
XIII. Paſtes of different Sorts.
XIV. Dried Conſerves.
XV. Of Cakes, Wafers, and Biſcuits.
XVI. Of Almonds and Piſtachios made
   in different Ways.
XVII. Marmalades.
XVIII. Jellies.
XIX. Liquid and dried Sweetmeats.
XX. Syrups and Brandy Fruits.
XXI. Ices, Ice Creams, and Ice Fruits.
XXII. Ratafias, and other Cordials, &c.

INCLUDING

A TRANSLATION of LES SOUPERS DE LA COUR;

WITH THE

Addition of the beſt Receipts which have ever appeared in the French or
Engliſh Languages, and adapted to the London Markets.

By B. CLERMONT,

Who has been many Years Clerk of the Kitchen in ſome of the firſt Families of this
Kingdom, and lately to the Right Hon. the Earl of ABINGDON.

The THIRD EDITION, reviſed and much enlarged.

LONDON:

Printed for W. DAVIS, in Piccadilly; T. CASLON, oppoſite Stationer's-Hall; G.
ROBINSON, in Paternoſter-Row; F. NEWBERY, the Corner of St. Paul's Church-
Yard; and the AUTHOR, in Princes-Street, Cavendiſh-Square.

M.DCC.LXXVI.

gives the Rich an opportunity of spending upon good Works, while they succour the Poor, and give comfort to them in their greatest Distresses.' Printed recipe collections could also be marketed as an alternative, or antidote, to the burdensome business of consulting professional doctors: as the author of *Natura Exenterata or Nature Unbowelled* (1655) claimed, he wished to help patients for whom *garrulus medicus est oneriosior morbo*, 'the wordy doctor is worse than the disease'.

The withdrawal of women

The second half of the seventeenth century saw women withdraw from the field of medical publication, as they did from medical practice in the wider world. Hannah Wolley claimed that though she had been 'Physitian and Chyurgeon in her own House to many … she dare not … adventure to teach but only those things wherein People cannot easily err' (preface to *The Queen-like Closet or Rich Cabinet … for Preserving, Candying and Cookery*, 1684). Printed works gradually shed most of their potentially controversial medical contents at the same time as they appealed more to a middling, less genteel readership. The engraved frontispiece to John Shirley's *The Accomplished Ladies Rich Closet of Rarities* (1691) shows a range of appropriate female household activities – nursing, distilling, dairying and so on – all safely distant from the paid activities of professional medical practitioners; while a title like *The Compleat Servant-Maid*, attributed to Hannah Wolley in 1685, indicates how the target audience for such publications was changing.

By the following century household books tend to be solidly middle-class in tone; their contents are dominated by cookery and related activities connected with diet; and their medicinal input is limited to the preparation of food for invalids, nursing the sick and the treatment of trivial childhood complaints.

MR BEETON'S SECRET

by Kathryn Hughes

It was January 2005 and I was nearing the end of writing my biography of Mrs Beeton, the Victorian cookery writer who died at the age of just 28. During the previous five years of research I'd been struck by the growing feeling that there was something more than bad luck underlying Isabella Beeton's run of miscarriages and sickly babies. Nor did the accepted wisdom that her husband Sam had suffered from consumption all his life before succumbing at the age of 46 quite add up.

By carefully sifting early family anecdotes it seemed increasingly likely to me that Sam had picked up syphilis from a prostitute when he was a bachelor and had passed on the disease to Isabella on her wedding night. This would explain her distressing inability to produce a thriving baby during the first seven years of her marriage. It would also make sense of the way that the final years of Sam's life were marked by dementia, a symptom associated with syphilis rather than TB.

But there was one problem with my theory. Earlier biographies, written mostly by members of the extended Beeton clan, always said that the consumptive Sam was tended by Dr Morrell MacKenzie, a society doctor who specialised in diseases of the throat and nose. I knew that throats and noses weren't quite the same as lungs, but still the fact that Sam was sent to a man who seemed to have no expertise in venereal disease suggested that my hunch was off.

In that first chilly week of 2005 I made one last effort to solve the mystery. I'd been told that MacKenzie's papers were in the Wellcome Library, although the first time I entered his name in the computer I drew a disappointing blank. It turned out that his name had been spelled incorrectly by the cataloguer, something which happened a great deal during his own lifetime. After much consultation with the librarian and some well-thumbed index cards, I finally established that the Wellcome did indeed hold some of MacKenzie's case notes for 1885. This was eight years after Sam Beeton had died, but still they would give me a sense of the kind of patients whom the good doctor habitually saw.

I couldn't believe what I found. There in MacKenzie's surprisingly careless hand was note after note describing the ravages of syphilis on his patients. There is poor Miss Hampson of Alnwick who is suffering from 'extensive ulceration of face' and unlucky Mr Steele whose symptoms started with a 'black scab at the end of nose', while Florence Carr, perhaps the worst case on his books, is dealing with 'destruction of nose which is flattened & the tip has fallen in entirely'. Elsewhere MacKenzie notes gloomily of this kind of nasal collapse, 'there is practically no limit to the ravages which may be committed by syphilis when once developed in this locality.'

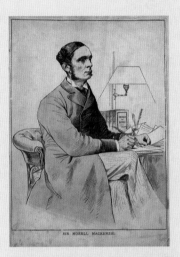

The nose and throat specialist and society doctor, Morrell MacKenzie, in 1888

So my hunch had been right after all! All the circumstantial evidence suggests that Sam Beeton was being treated by Morrell MacKenzie not on account of his lungs but because his throat, and possibly his nose too, was ravaged by the effects of end stage syphilis. Of course, until Sam's actual case notes turn up, we can never be certain. Which means, in turn, that it is impossible to be definite about Isabella losing all those unborn and sickly babies to this horrible disease. But, until that moment of certainty comes, I'm happy to rest my case.

❖

IMPACTS OF

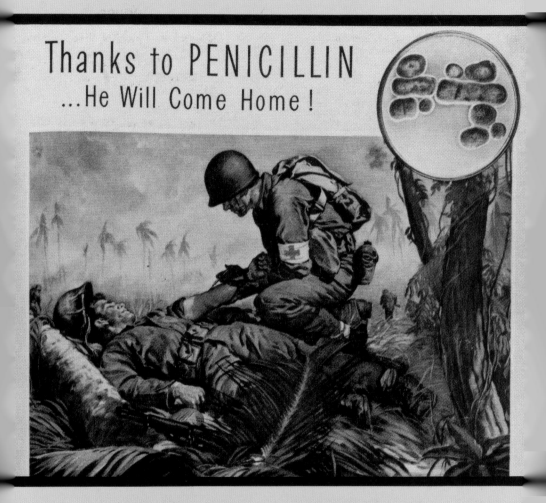

Thanks to PENICILLIN

...He Will Come Home!

ANTIBIOTIC-RESISTANT BACTERIA

3
BREAKTHROUGHS AND BUST-UPS: EXPERIMENTS AND DISCOVERIES IN MODERN MEDICINE

Nowadays medical breakthroughs are rarely the work of a single person; rather they are the result of research by international teams. Hard work and careful planning, as well as fate and luck, all play their part in discoveries, as scientists themselves acknowledge. Yet the challenge to be first to publish results remains paramount. Individual claims to fame may be just one of several issues that make us turn to the records and personal papers of medical scientists, but it's one that features largely in both the penicillin and the DNA story.

Penicillin and the discovery of the structure of DNA were both triumphs for British researchers and led to the award of Nobel prizes to key players. These stories of discovery have much in common. Inevitably there is the shared scenario of what *might* have happened had things been done differently, had an observation been made by a different person at a different time. Other common factors are the presence of individual scientists with incredible determination and strong beliefs, fraught relationships between team workers and other scientists in the field, the importance of competition in spurring researchers to find the answers, the significance of the publication of results, issues around who was credited with the discoveries, and the fact that not all those closely involved were rewarded with public recognition. Francis Crick and James Watson won Nobels in 1962 for their work on DNA, but many believe that Rosalind Franklin's work should also have been honoured (though her early death rendered her ineligible for a Nobel). Alexander Fleming, Howard Florey and Ernst Chain gained Nobels in 1945 for their role in the discovery of penicillin, but, arguably, the role played by Norman Heatley has been underestimated.

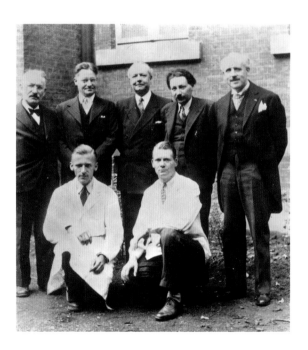

Previous page:
A US Second World War poster extolling the benefits of penicillin in jungle warfare

Left:
Group portrait of scientists at the William Dunn School of Pathology, Oxford. Howard Florey is second from the left in the back row, and Ernst Chain is second from the right

A 'top ten' list of discoveries and
achievements in medical treatment
during the twentieth century might
look something like this:

– the discovery of sulphonamides (1935)
– the discovery of penicillin (1941)
– the cure for tuberculosis with streptomycin
  and PAS (1950)
– the discovery of the molecular structure
  of DNA (1953)
– the oral contraceptive pill (1960)
– Charnley's hip replacement surgery (1961)
– kidney transplantation (1963)
– the CAT scanner (1973)
– the discovery of embryonic stem cells (1981)
– the 'sequencing' of DNA (1998)

The Wellcome Library holds archives
and publications which tell us about these
and many other major developments
in medical science.

The story of the discovery of penicillin starts with Alexander
Fleming's research and his chance discovery of a fungal contaminant
(named *Penicillium notatum*) that grew on a plate left in his laboratory
at St Mary's Hospital, London. Fleming's work on treating wound
infections enabled him to recognise the importance of the mould
and how it could be used. This happened in 1929, and whilst the
effectiveness of the antibiotic was soon understood, several more
years would pass before other scientists discovered how to produce
penicillin on an industrial scale. Howard Florey, working at the
William Dunn School of Pathology, Oxford, managed to cultivate
the fungus, assisted by Norman Heatley. Ernst Chain was also
there and initially worked with them, later helping develop mass
production. Penicillin remains a front-line antibiotic in common
use for bacterial infections and has saved millions of lives.

We all know that when we compose a paper
setting out ... discoveries we write it in such
a way that the planning and unfolding of the
experiments appear to be a beautiful and logical
sequence, but we all know that the facts are that
we usually blunder from one lot of dubious
observations to another and only at the end do we
see how we should have set about our problems.

From Howard Florey's Dunham Lectures, 1965

A bit of a boffin

Norman Heatley (1911–2004) was a research biochemist and he was responsible for carrying out many of the technical innovations that were used in the complex processes of extracting and purifying penicillin and measuring its activity. It was Heatley's monitoring of experiments on mice that first showed the therapeutic potential of penicillin and his development of a reliable yet simple assay method for penicillin, which was crucial. His small but highly significant collection was given by him to the Wellcome Library, and following his death additional papers and diaries were given by his family.[1] They contain laboratory notebooks from October 1939 to June 1941 when he was doing his vital research at the Dunn School. The famous experiment of 25 May 1941 on 'the curative effect of penicillin on mice' is recorded in notebook A.2. There are also diary entries, narratives and explanatory notes, as well as notes expressly written by Heatley to accompany his papers.

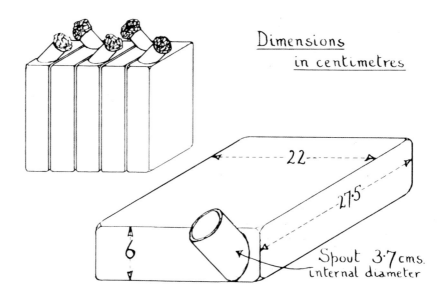

Norman Heatley's design of ceramic vessels for culturing penicillin, to be specially manufactured by James Macintyre & Co. Ltd, Burslem, 1940

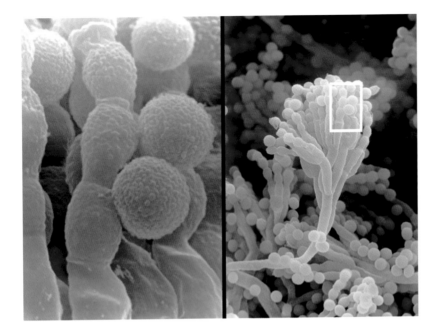

Scanning electron micrograph of *Penicillium* mould-producing spores, with (at far left) close-up of spore formation, 2003

Heatley was a bit of a 'boffin'. He had a marvellous gift for conjuring up equipment during wartime shortages, and he was clearly proud of the use he made of a large number of discarded squash bottles, for example, which were fortuitously acquired by the laboratory. These could be adapted for a number of purposes. A small hole was drilled near the bottom and with further modifications they were used to extract and purify penicillin, which at first proved difficult to do. Milk churns, hospital bedpans, biscuit tins and pie dishes were all pressed into service to help with the culture of penicillin before custom-made ceramic dishes were acquired from the Potteries.

The idea of using back-extraction to separate and produce penicillin was to become a source of serious controversy between Chain, Heatley and Florey. In a discussion between all three in March 1940, Heatley suggested a method which took advantage of the solubility of penicillin in ether or chloroform. Chain thought it would not work and dismissed the idea. Florey supported Heatley's desire to try and see. So Heatley made the first trial and proved the feasibility of his method (a back-extraction process using amyl acetate), which was to be the basis of commercial production.

The episode was one of several disagreements between the three scientists. Ernst Chain (1906–79) had left Berlin in 1933; his mother and sister would both disappear without trace during the Second World War. Among the 69 boxes placed in the Wellcome by his family, there is one section with reports, correspondence and notes and accounts of penicillin research.[2] Chain came across Fleming's work on penicillin as part of his larger research with Florey into antibiotics and enzymes. Sadly, there are no notebooks and few records of the actual experiments conducted, and most of the information about this work is found in later correspondence, notes for talks and historical accounts.

Chain's version of the 1940 discussion differs from his colleagues'. He believed that they were trespassing on his domain, which was the chemical side of the work. He bore a grudge for the rest of his life and his papers include notes vindicating himself. Interestingly, a previous collaboration between Chain and Heatley in 1936 had already shown that they were 'somewhat allergic to each other', as Ronald Clarke puts it in *The Life of Ernst Chain* (1985).

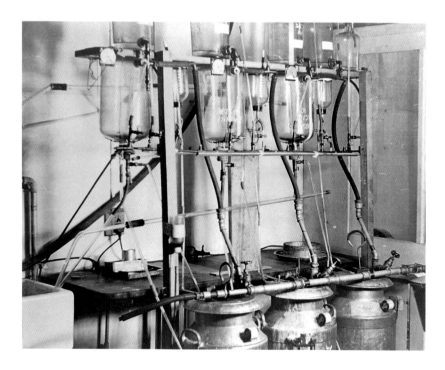

Milk churns and other equipment used in the early production of penicillin (1940–41)

In his papers Chain comes across as a determined and forceful character with a love of music, strong family ties and support for Jewish organisations. He could be combative and touchy, and was certainly not a 'clubbable' man, though he resented not being accepted as a member of the Athenaeum as were Florey and Fleming.

When the first paper on penicillin came to be published no individual credit for particular work was assigned to the scientists involved. The Nobel prize was awarded to Fleming, Florey and Chain in 1945, but relations between Florey and Chain were very strained and both men resented Fleming's claims, which they felt went too far. Heatley, meanwhile, had to wait years for public recognition. He was awarded an OBE for his contribution to scientific research in 1978 and given the first honorary Doctorate of Medicine ever conferred by Oxford University in 1990.

Crick and DNA

The excitement generated by the Wellcome Trust's purchase of the papers of Francis Crick (1916–2004) in 2001, with assistance from the Heritage Lottery Fund, is evidence of their exceptional importance. Crick's scientific contribution has been compared to that of Newton. The collection covers all his working papers, but this description belies the very personal nature of some of the material, since they, like Chain's papers, include correspondence with many eminent scientists and organisations on a wide range of topics.[3] Again like Chain, Crick had presence and a strong personality. He was eloquent (his endless chatter and loud laugh could sometimes irritate colleagues) and was in great demand as a speaker. His later career demonstrates that his ability to inspire and influence was as important, if not more important, than the research he was then doing, which from the 1980s shifted into theoretical work in neurobiology, particularly consciousness.

All we had to work on were certain fragmentary experimental results, themselves often uncertain and confused, and a boundless optimism that the basic concepts involved were rather simple and probably much the same in all living things. In such a situation well constructed theories can play a really useful part in stating problems clearly and thus guiding experiment.

Francis Crick, 'Central dogma of molecular biology', *Nature*, 227, p. 561

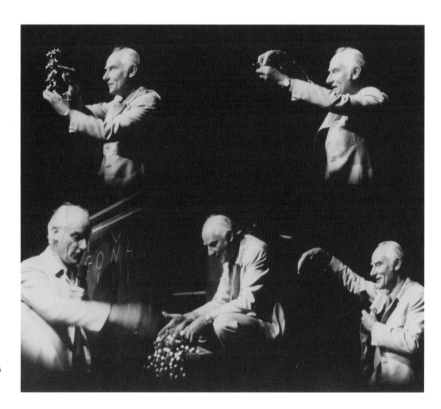

A composite photo of Francis Crick lecturing on DNA, by Bradley Smith, 1976

each one set off bursts of hypotheses, theories, suggestions for investigation in his mind … the experience was like sitting next to an intellectual nuclear reactor … I have never had a feeling of such incandescence.

Oliver Sachs, 'Remembering Francis Crick', *New York Review of Books*, 24 March 2005

From:
M.R.C., *Laboratory of Molecular Biology, Hills Road, Cambridge.*

Dr. F. H. C. Crick thanks you for your letter but regrets that he is unable to accept your kind invitation to:

send an autograph	read your manuscript
provide a photograph	deliver a lecture
cure your disease	attend a conference
be interviewed	act as chairman
talk on the radio	become an editor
appear on TV	contribute an article
speak after dinner	write a book
give a testimonial	accept an honorary degree
help you in your project	

The price of fame: Francis Crick's multi-purpose reply card, dating from the 1960s

Crick's keen intellect was matched by his wit, charm and mischievous nature. He worked best in collaboration with close colleagues, each firing ideas at the other. His impact on the public was so great that he was besieged by letters from fans and requests for autographs, though he rather shunned fame and publicity. He therefore devised a postcard consisting of standard replies and would simply tick the relevant box. Some correspondents appeared to expect him to be able to solve all problems, as though he were a miracle worker. His responses could be terse and sarcastic. He famously resigned his Fellowship at Churchill College, Cambridge, when they threatened to build a college chapel, and suggested that the money might as well be used to provide a college brothel. But he could also be very considerate and was more than willing to give time to people and causes he thought worthy of it. Encouraging children to take an interest in science was one such cause and – right up to the late 1990s – he continued to accept invitations to lecture to schools when he was refusing all other engagements.

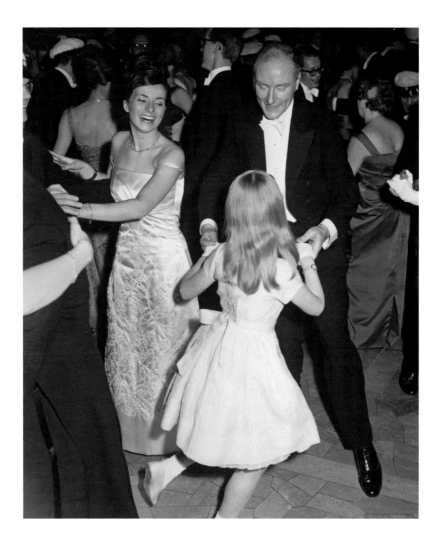

Francis Crick with his wife Odile and daughter Gabrielle at the Nobel banquet, Stockholm, 1962

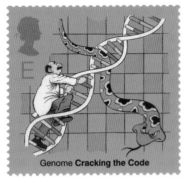

Genome **Cracking the Code**

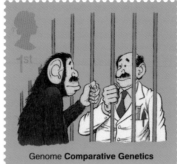

Genome **Comparative Genetics**

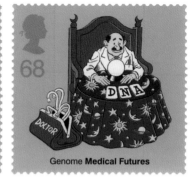

Genome **Medical Futures**

Crick worked at the Cavendish Laboratory in Cambridge with Max Perutz and John Kendrew, investigating the structure of proteins through X-ray crystallography. James Watson joined the laboratory in 1951, and the two men developed their interest in identifying the structure of genetic material, drawing on the experimental data produced at King's College, London, by Rosalind Franklin and Maurice Wilkins. They were well aware of the significance of their proposed double-helical structure of DNA, an essential step in the discovery of the transmission of genetic information. Yet the famous first paper in *Nature* (25 April 1953) contained the great understatement that 'it has not escaped our notice that the specific pairing [of purine and pyrimidine bases] that we have postulated immediately suggests a possible copying mechanism for the genetic material'. Crick and Watson had debated the wording. While Watson was cautious about making a claim that might not be supported, Crick was all for claiming priority, for fear that if they failed to point out the potential significance others might think they were unaware of it.

Debate continues over whether Crick and Watson acted insensitively in the way they used information from Rosalind Franklin. Franklin does not seem to have borne a grudge, and indeed she was to become a good friend of Crick's before her early death in 1958, aged 37. Watson's bestselling book, *The Double Helix* (1968), fuelled the debate and upset many of the key players, including Crick, who – at first, at least – felt that Watson had so debased their

Royal Mail stamps celebrating the 50th anniversary of the discovery of the structure of DNA, 2003

achievement with his gossipy superficial account that 'it sounded as if anybody could have done it'. As always, personality differences and misunderstandings played a large part in the tensions, and certainly many other scientists contributed to the discovery of the double helix apart from Crick and Watson, including Wilkins, Linus Pauling and Erwin Chargaff, as well as Franklin.

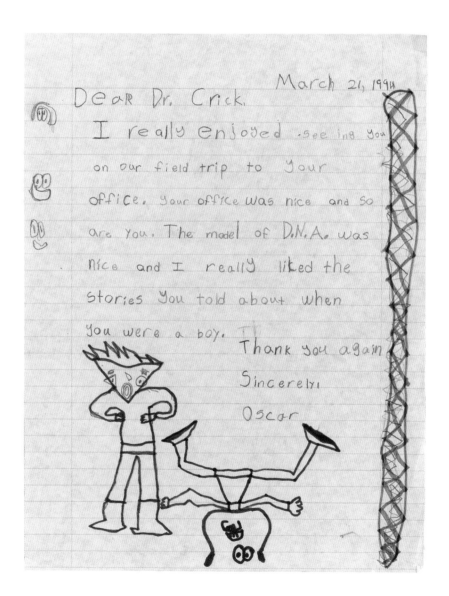

A child's thank-you letter to Crick following a school visit to his office in 1994, complete with drawing of Crick and of the double helix. Crick kept Oscar's letter among his papers

THE ROVING INTELLECT
OF FRANCIS CRICK
by Robert Olby

M y first experience of working on Dr Crick's papers must have been in 1990 when he agreed to my suggestion to write his biography. That meant trips to the Salk Institute in La Jolla. Many a time I climbed the staircase beside the Salk Institute library and emerged onto a long wood-panelled corridor at the far end of which Crick's personal assistant, Maria Lang, had her desk – as did her successor, Kathleen Murray. To the left was Crick's spacious office and to right and left were ante-rooms filled with what are now the Crick papers at the Wellcome.[1] Lining one side of the corridor was a series of box files containing a multitude of correspondence marked 'refusals' that Crick liked to point out with evident amusement. Working on the papers there was idyllic, but for the absence of any finding aids.

Originally Crick favoured my suggestion that his papers be deposited at the University of California at San Diego. Lynda Claassen, UCSD's Archives Director, was enthusiastic, but then came the suggestion that the papers be sold to Mr Jeremy Norman, the rare book and archive dealer in California, with an interest in scientific archives. Characteristically, Crick asked his lawyer to look into the proposed deal. There were problems, and at that point Dr James Watson turned to the Wellcome Trust, advising them to step in. How wise he was. Since then it has been wonderful to see the collection growing, to have the masterful guide prepared by Chris Beckett and continued by his successors, and always the helpful assistance of the archives staff.

There are many features of the Francis Crick papers that make the collection a very precious resource. Foremost, naturally, is the personality of Crick. His roving intellect and intense curiosity took him into many a corner of science and beyond to solve fundamental problems in biology. Take the genetic code. To its solution Crick brought data from the plant viruses, their structure, chemical constitution and mutation, from the genetics and mutability of bacteriophages, from the stereochemistry of the amino acids, proteins, and ribonucleic acids, and from cryptography. To follow adequately the thread leading to the discovery of the genetic code one needs to research all these subject areas, for the direct approach to the code via protein synthesis in the test tube – 'the cell-free system' – was not achieved until eight years after the discovery of the structure of DNA. Meanwhile all these indirect approaches were attempted. Fortunately they are all represented in the collection because Crick kept the relevant correspondence with the notes and drafts of his talks.

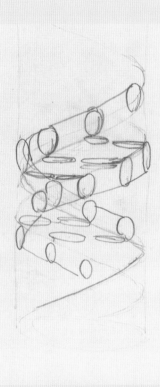

Crick's pencil sketch of the DNA double helix from 1953

From this archive we can also chart the spread of the new knowledge as Crick attended meetings, symposia, congresses and summer schools, at first in the USA and the UK, but year by year in more and more countries, until his doctor began advising him to take a complete rest. This activity took its toll, for he was not at these events just for the ride. Nor would he just give his talk and be quiet. He would provoke, cajole, rebut and persuade, as we can see from the discussions at these meetings.

At one moment he was the theoretician of X-ray crystallographic methods who perceived the strengths and limitations of Patterson analysis, the power of model building, and the theory of the method of isomorphous replacement. The issues involved found a lively place in his long-standing debates with the incorrigible sceptic, Jerry Donohue. At another time he was developing with James Watson the crystallographic principles of the structure of viruses. Fascination with molecular evolution drew him with Leslie Orgel to the origin of life and the origin of the genetic code. The mystery of embryological development caused him to study insect development with Peter Lawrence and chromosome structure with Roger Kornberg and Sir Aaron Klug. These were topics ripe for investigation with the new understanding of genes and their template role in protein synthesis. Thus can we view the activity of 'going molecular' in biology through the window of its foremost protagonist.

Another feature of the collection is the element of amusement stemming from the controversial nature of many of Crick's claims. Crick sought to educate a general audience about molecular biology through his John Danz Lectures (*Molecules and Men*), his imaginative little book on the origin of life (*Life Itself*) and his autobiography (*What Mad Pursuit*). In *The Astonishing Hypothesis* he aimed to disabuse those who believe in an afterlife by teaching them neuroscience. The files contain many amusing responses to these works, such as 'Does he need the money that badly?' In view of his atheistic pronouncements one smart alec displayed the one-liner, 'Crick for God.' Crick's attack on the arts in *Molecules and Men* was described by one reviewer as 'conquest by violence'. Another complained that reductionism in this book is 'enthroned in biology as some sort of religious dogma'.

When in his sixties Crick turned to neuroscience, he had as his long-term goal to confront the mystery of consciousness. But his plan was to approach this subject from within neuroscience, not from outside it. This meant learning the existing science first. He would as usual teach himself, but also he would invite neuroscientists to the Salk Institute and have intensive discussions with them. His strategy was to explore the several approaches – hence the archives have correspondence with computationists in artificial intelligence, David Marr, Christopher Longuet-Higgins, Tomaso Poggio, Valentino Braitenberg and the mathematician Graeme Mitchison. At the same time he was continuing to follow David Hubel's work in neurophysiology, for it was the Hubel/Wiesel study of the functional anatomy of the visual system that had so impressed him in the 1960s. The result of all these skirmishes into new territories is an archive wide-ranging in its subject matter and fascinating.

Last but not least, is the wealth of jokes, asides hiding between the lines, the abiding sense of fun, good humour and from time to time stern words turning occasionally to rage. Just to take one example of fun: Rose Feiner's verse about Crick's wobble hypothesis. It was rejected by *Nature*, but she sent it to Crick:

On a ribosome unit a messenger sat
Singing 'wobble, O wobble, O wobble';
And I said to a codon, 'O why do you sit
Singing wobble, O wobble, O wobble?

Is it weakness of Watson your little inside
Or a Crick in your intercistronic divide?'
With a flip of a hydrogen bond it replied
'O wobble, O wobble, O wobble!'[2]

❖

حصل تأسيس مدرسة الطب بأبى زعبل على يد رئيسها الشهير كلوت بيك فى شهر ذى الحجة الحرام سنة ١٢٤٢

مجد العلوم فى الديار المصرية حضرة الداورى الاعظم افندينا ولى النعم محمد على باشا

وكان انتقالها من ابى زعبل الى مصر المحروسة فى غرة محرم سنة ١٢٥٣ هجرية

بسم الله الرحمن الرحيم

هذا عهد الاطباء

اقسم بالله العظيم ❀ وبنبيه الكريم ❀ محمد صلى الله عليه وسلم ❀ على أنى أكون أمينا حريصا على شروط الشرف والبر والصلاح ❀ فى تعاطى صناعة الطب ❀ وأن أسعف الفقراء مجانا ❀ ولا اطلب اجرة تزيد عن اجرة عملى ❀ وانى اذا دخلت بيتا فلا تنظر عيناى ما ذا يحصل فيه ❀ ولا ينطق لسانى بالأسرار التى يأتمنونى عليها ❀ ولا استعمل صناعتى فى افساد الخصال الحميدة ❀ ولا اعاون بها على الذنوب ❀ ولا اعطى سما البتة ولا ادل عليه ولا اشيره ❀ ولا اعطى دواء فيه ضرر على الحوامل ولا اسقاطهن ❀ واكون موقرا وحافظا للمعروف مع الذين علمونى ❀ ومكافئا الأولاد هم بتعليمى اياهم ما تعلمته من آبائهم فما دمت حريصا على عهدى ❀ وأمينا على يمينى ❀ فجميع الناس يعتبرونى ويوقرونى ❀ وان خالفت ذلك فأكون المرذل المحتقر والله الشهيد على ما اقوله ❀

طبع بالمطبعة الطبية الدرنه هدية من صاحبها هذه المطبعة لتلامذة المدرسة الطبية

4
A CARD WRITTEN IN ARABIC: AN ORIENTAL TALE

The *Oriens Extremus* and *Oriens Proximus* (nowadays Asia, Africa and Oceania) take pride of place in the Wellcome Library. Manuscript books in Arabic and Turkish, Sanskrit and Burmese, as well as Hebrew scrolls and Syriac parchments, manuscripts on palm leaves and birch bark, comprise the medical wisdom of the peoples of the East. This wisdom was directly connected to the individuals who created and transmitted it. Along with sages and physicians there are the scribes who recorded it and the illuminators and binders who adorned and protected the neatly written pages. In almost every instance the history of an oriental manuscript and its provenance is as interesting as the text itself. Modern readers can enjoy the fruits of the labour of Buddhist monks and Chinese silk-weavers who created masterpieces in the art of the book. They can admire the attempts of a mediaeval Syrian scribe to protect his ownership of a rare manuscript and relish the derogatory remark of an eighteenth-century Indian intellectual criticising an incomplete Arabic text. Even a piece of cardboard can have an intriguing history.

In the spring of 1905 a mysterious 'card written in Arabic' arrived at the London headquarters of Burroughs Wellcome & Co. from Cairo.[1] Neither Henry S. Wellcome, who had been collecting artefacts for a 'Historical Medical Exhibition' that was originally planned for 1904, nor his secretaries could read the oriental script. In acknowledging its receipt Wellcome wrote to the donor, Dr Mohammed Nashed: 'I did not answer your letter earlier because I was expecting a translation. If it does not overburden you, would it be possible to submit it?'[2] Dr Nashed, who taught in the Kasr al-Ayni medical school between 1883 and 1889, clearly failed to produce the requested translation on time, because the 'card' was eventually translated into English in London and, when its contents

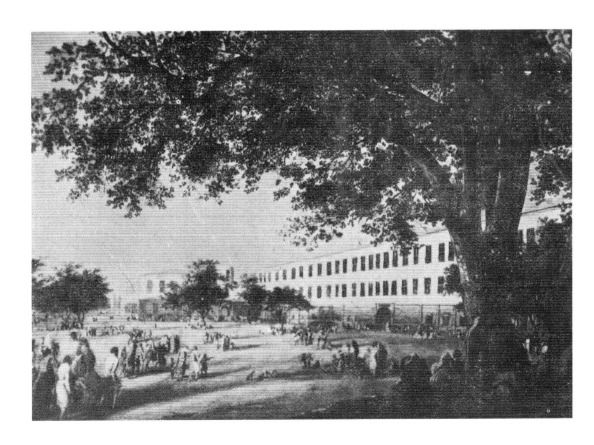

were known, another letter of thanks duly despatched to Cairo. But this translation was subsequently lost and the 'card' itself, for some unknown reason, relegated to the stacks.

On examination the card turned out to be a special edition of an oath sworn by the medical students of the Kasr al-Ayni medical school. It was printed and donated to the students to commemorate the fiftieth anniversary in 1883 of the school's transfer to Kasr al-Ayni from Abu Zaabal, the place where it had been founded. The text of the oath in fact has very little to do with Arab and Islamic medical traditions, but owes a great deal to the activities of a Frenchman, Antoine Barthélémy Clot-Bey (1793–1868). A medical practitioner, prolific writer and an entrepreneur, Antoine Barthélémy Clot was famous for organising the first medical school in Egypt, as well as for being the first Catholic to be decorated with the title Bey (literally 'master', the nineteenth-century Arabic equivalent of an English knighthood) for combating the plague.

Clot-Bey did not have an easy life. The son of a sergeant-major in the Napoleonic army, he received his initial medical training under his father's comrade, Mr Sapey, a retired army surgeon. The first operation he performed was for the removal of a sebaceous cyst, which he preserved in alcohol and carried with him as a memento for many years. In 1813 he set out for Marseille, where a fellow medical student helped him gain entry to the Hôtel-Dieu, the city hospital. Clot succeeded in passing the entrance exams and was not only admitted as a student *externe* but was considered to be the best. His degree in medicine did not, however, bring him enough means to support his widowed mother. Further years of study, first at the University of Aix-en-Provence and then at the medical school in Montpellier, were required before he was made assistant surgeon at the Hôtel-Dieu in Marseille. After his return to Montpellier in 1823 to present his thesis for an MD in surgery, he was dropped from the Academic Society of Medicine of Marseille and banned from giving lessons in the hospitals there, probably out of envy of his success.

Surgeon-in-Chief of the Egyptian Army

Two years later Clot-Bey's life was transformed when he entered the service of Muhammad Ali, the Ottoman viceroy of Egypt, who was concerned about the health of his army. Clot-Bey was made the Surgeon-in-Chief of the Armies and immediately introduced French army health regulations in the Egyptian army camps. He convinced Muhammad Ali that the way to keep the army healthy was to raise the standard of health in the general population and make smallpox vaccination mandatory for civilians. He founded a medical school for 300 students at the 1,500-bed military hospital at Abu Zaabal, which was located outside Cairo. Initially he commissioned European doctors to teach there, but his aim in founding the school was eventually to replace them with local personnel. In this he faced two major obstacles – language and religious opposition.

He solved the first problem by introducing an institute of interpreters. The second was more difficult to tackle: there was even an attempt to kill Clot-Bey while he was giving an anatomy demonstration. But he appealed to the religious authorities, the ūlema', saying that by studying medicine they would increase their influence; consequently several ūlema' themselves became medical students and one of them even composed a medical dictionary. Clot-Bey assuaged their objections by making concessions to the Muslim religion. He selected the holy month of Ramadan as the major holiday for the medical school, which was soon teaching four different curricula: human and veterinary medicine, pharmacy and midwifery. In 1830 he organised a very successful public examination for his students, bringing in an outside examiner from Europe. In less than five years Clot-Bey had managed to set up a western-style medical school and produce Egyptian students capable of competing with their European counterparts.

The Frenchman
Antoine Barthélémy Clot
(Clot-Bey), founder of the
first medical school in Egypt

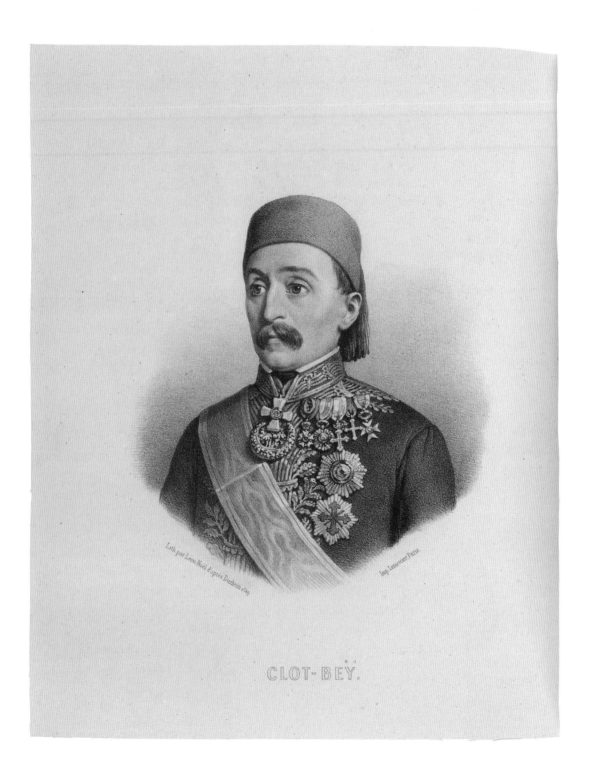

CLOT-BEY.

Lith. par Leon-Noël d'après Durheim 1849

Imp. Lemercier, Paris.

The Hippocratic Oath – Oriental-style

Like every other such establishment Clot-Bey's medical school required an ethos, which in this case was based on the nineteenth-century European tradition of the so-called 'Hippocratic Oath'. In fact the oath ascribed to Hippocrates, the 'Father of Medicine', who lived c. 460–380 BC on the Greek island of Cos, was introduced in Western Europe rather late: the first recorded use of it is in 1508 in the University of Wittenberg (Germany), a university famous for its classical and humanist traditions. It did not become a standard part of a French medical school graduation ceremony until 1804, when it was incorporated into the commencement exercises at Montpellier. As an alumnus of Montpellier himself, Clot-Bey had the ingenious idea of adapting the Hippocratic Oath to the needs of an Islamic medical institution. There were legitimate grounds for this: Hippocrates (or 'Buqrat' in Arabic) enjoyed a high reputation in the Arab Islamic medical tradition: his name was mentioned even in proverbs. As a physician, he was esteemed by dozens of Arab doctors, among them such luminaries as Avicenna and Rhazes. The Arabic translation of the 'Oath' was not unknown to educated Arabs; it was even cited in full in the famous *History of Doctors* written by the thirteenth-century physician, Ibn Abi Usaibi'a (1203–70).

Still, Clot-Bey and his advisers had to adapt it to local conditions. In the new variant a Muslim doctor did not have to swear by the Greek pagan gods Apollo, Asclepius, Hygieia and Panaceia, as did his contemporary French colleague. Instead he swore in the name of the Most High God and His Messenger, the Prophet Muhammad. Ancient Greek rules regarding the relationship between master and student also had to be changed. A Muslim doctor did not promise to hold his teacher 'as equal' to his parents. Nor did he swear 'to live his life in partnership with him, and if he is in need of money to give him a share of mine, and to regard his offspring as equal to his brothers in male lineage and to teach them this art – if they desire to learn it – without fee and covenant'. The responsibilities of a Muslim doctor were more limited: 'Ever respectful and grateful to my masters, I will hand on to their children the instruction which I had received from their fathers.'

Similarly, the Muslim version excluded the original paragraphs about applying dietetic measures for the benefit of the sick. But the promise 'to keep the patients away from harm and injustice' was precisely specified: 'I will attend the poor gratuitously, and will never exact too high a fee for my work.' The Hippocratic undertaking not to give anybody a deadly drug, or administer to a woman an abortive remedy, was kept more or less intact: 'I will neither give nor prescribe to any pregnant woman dangerous drugs capable of provoking or producing an abortion.'

The Hippocratic Oath originally contained two other important statements regarding the abuse of a physician's position:

> Whatever houses I may visit, I will come for the benefit of the sick, remaining free of all intentional injustice, of all mischief and in particular of sexual relations with both female and male persons, be they free or slaves. What I may see or hear in the course of the treatment or even outside of the treatment in regard to the life of men, which on no account one must spread abroad, I will keep to myself, holding such things shameful to be spoken about.

In the Muslim variant such specific injunctions were omitted and the whole idea was reduced to a generalised exhortation: 'admitted into the privacy of a house, my eyes will not perceive what takes place therein; my tongue will guard the secret confided to me. My art shall not serve to corrupt, nor to assist crime.'

The text of the Muslim oath was not available in the west until 1935, when a translation of it was published in the *History of Medical Education in Egypt* by the renowned Egyptian obstetrician Naguib Mikhail Pasha Mahfouz (1882–1974). (An unborn child whose life Naguib Mahfouz preserved when he treated the very sick mother at the time of the boy's birth in 1911 was named after him in gratitude and grew up to give that name the added lustre of a Nobel prize for literature.) But the number of copies of the doctor's book, printed in Cairo, was limited and this interesting document remained almost totally unknown beyond the banks of Nile, as did Clot-Bey's achievement in transforming the archaic Hippocratic Oath into a modern, practical code for Egyptian doctors.

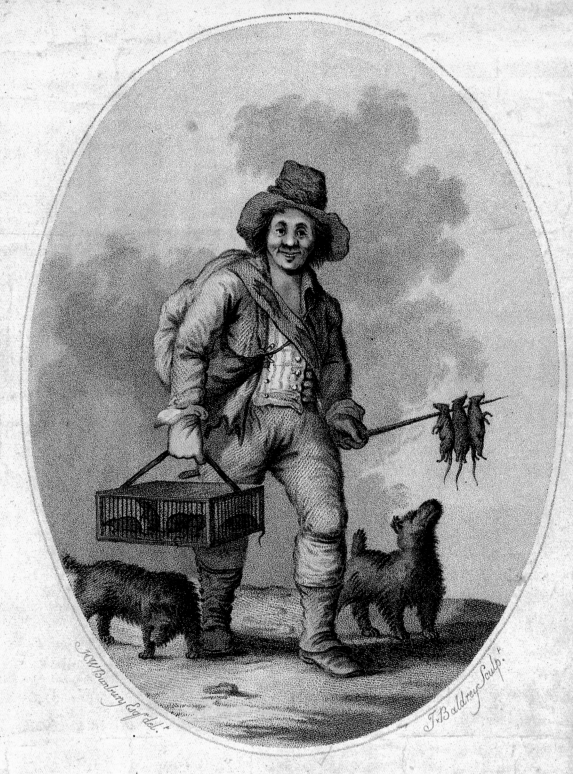

H. W. Bunbury Esq.r del.t

T. Baldrey Sculp.t

A Rat-Catcher.

London Publish.d Jan.ry 26. 1789. by W. Dickinson New Bond Street.

5
PLAGUES, PESTS AND POLLUTION: PUBLIC HEALTH AND ITS CUSTODIANS

The concept of 'Public Health' emerged in Britain in the 1830s and 1840s at a time of growing city populations, increasing urban squalor and rising levels of infectious disease, problems that government investigators began to address in the late 1830s. The 1848 Public Health Act required local authorities in towns with death rates of more than 23 per 1,000 inhabitants to appoint suitably qualified Medical Officers of Health (MOsH) whose job was to discover, investigate and control local sources of disease. But it was not until the passing of the 1872 Public Health Act, when each of the 1,400 sanitary districts into which England and Wales had been divided was obliged to appoint an MOH, that the country acquired a national public health system.

From the start all Medical Officers of Health were required to compile annual reports. The extensive collection of these reports in the Wellcome Library – over 2,800 of them – provides a continuous record of public health activity across the country and is one of the richest available sources on local public health administration, patterns of disease, social conditions and public and personal behaviour in the years between about 1850 and 1974. The collection includes a wide variety of English, Welsh and Scottish reports for both urban and rural districts, county boroughs and counties, as well as metropolitan vestries and boroughs. There are also reports by two occupational sub-groups, the Port Medical Officers, appointed from 1872, and the School Medical Officers, from 1907, on the establishment of the School Medical Services.

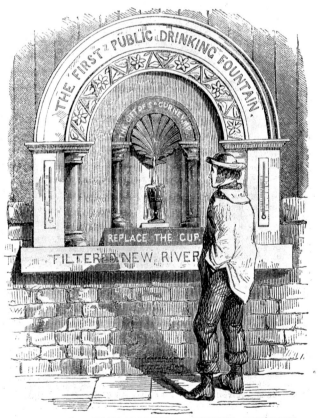

THE FIRST LONDON DRINKING FOUNTAIN, ADJOINING
ST. SEPULCHRE'S CHURCH, SNOW HILL.

Previous page:
An engraving from
1789 of a rat-catcher
displaying the fruits
of his labour

Left:
London's first drinking
fountain, 1858

Do you know the Medical Officer of Health for your parish? 'I never see him,' you say. How do you think your parish is kept in good health? How do you think that the water supply of London is kept as perfect as that of any other town in the world? No other large city in the world can say there is an absence of typhoid fever. Who sees that the milk and meat supplies are in good condition? The Medical Officer of Health. 'I didn't know that before.' Are your drains in good condition? The Medical Officer of Health sees to that too; he goes into your house and examines it. … This, then, is our hope for the future, this great Department of Public Health, this great Department of Officers of Health all over the country.

From a draft sermon by Sir James Cantlie, President of the Royal Society of Tropical Medicine and Hygiene, c. 1920[1]

What is in the MOH Reports?

Between 1850 and 1900 the focus of the MOH reports is largely on infectious diseases, housing, water supplies, sewers and drains, nuisances and refuse disposal. There are detailed accounts of infectious diseases as they affect local districts – smallpox, typhoid and typhus, cholera, scarlet fever, diphtheria, measles, whooping cough and diarrhoea; sometimes respiratory tuberculosis and bronchitis. You will find figures of annual deaths and descriptions of outbreaks. There may be information on a wide range of local problems, from the nuisance of urban pig-keeping, through pickle manufacturers and fish fryers and cats' meat processors, to the disposal of horse manure and the amount of straw that some hospitals would put down in the streets to deaden traffic noise for their patients.

The quality of the reports varies, depending mostly on the character and dedication of the MOH in question. Some reports are brief, not much more than leaflets; others are long and extremely rich, like those of T. Orme Dudfield at Kensington, of John Tripe at Hackney and John Syer Bristowe at Camberwell in nineteenth-century London. Bristowe describes, for example, the small house of a costermonger who – not unusually – kept two donkeys and a clutch of rabbits in one of the downstairs rooms, and at least a hundred ducks and fowls in two of the upstairs bedrooms, the floors being 'thick with their filth'. In the provinces, the reports for Birmingham and Manchester stand out for quality of writing and information contained, but there are many others that are as valuable. Those for Port Health Authorities have their own particular concerns, including emigration, infectious diseases brought in by passengers or crew, sanitation of vessels and the ubiquitous 'Rat problem'.

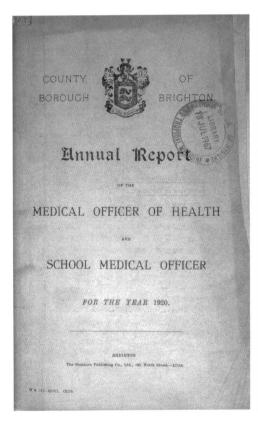

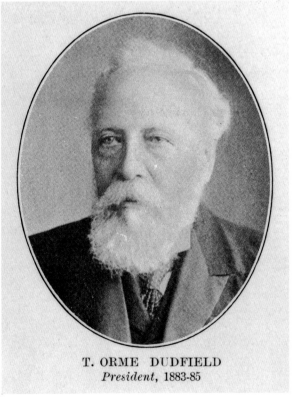

T. ORME DUDFIELD
President, 1883-85

Outside medical circles, the extent of these corroding cankers which live upon our social system is scarcely known; gonorrhea helps to fill the blind asylums with children infected at birth with ophthalmia, it provides women's hospitals with a considerable proportion of their patients, and causes years of suffering to those women who have been infected with the diseases. But, though gonorrhea in its various manifestations is potent for evil, yet it is not so terrible a disease as syphilis, the effects of which dog the patient for dozens of years, cause his children to be born dead, or, if they survive, to be tainted with disease and often struck down by blindness, deafness or mental weakness during childhood or adolescence; while not infrequently, years after the infection, the unhappy man loses his reason and dies in an asylum. About one-fifth of the patients who die in the Lancashire Asylums have their deaths certified to be due to general paralysis, which is now known to be almost always, if not absolutely always, a result of syphilis.

From Bootle MOH Report by (William) Allen Daley, 1913

Far left:
The title page of the 1920 Annual Report of the MOH and School Medical Officer for Brighton

Near left:
The Kensington MOH, T. Orme Dudfield, c.1885

IF YOU
FIND
DIRT
AT THE
BOTTOM

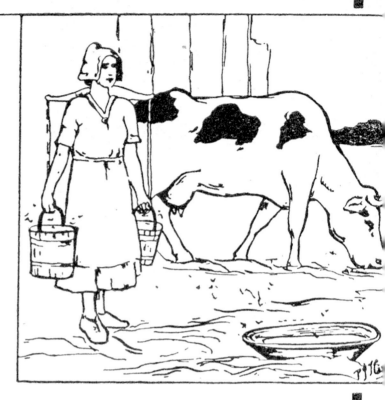

OF YOUR MILK JUG

TELL YOUR

Medical Officer of Health

AND COMPLAIN TO YOUR

MILKMAN.

The domestic and the personal

The end of the nineteenth century brings a change in emphasis in the MOH reports. On the one hand there is evidence of a more scientific approach to disease prevention; on the other, a shift of interest away from the infectious diseases, into the domestic and the personal. Women sanitary inspectors and health visitors began to be appointed in order to gain access to homes and educate women in hygiene and child care. This new focus on the home and on the care of infants and children was encouraged by powerful political factors: the twin spectres of physical deterioration and of a falling birth rate, both of which assumed alarming proportions when viewed through the lens of a prospective war against Germany. Britain's defeats in the Boer War had lent a sharp edge to these concerns and social legislation began to address these issues.

One outcome was the establishment of the School Medical Service. (William) Allen Daley's 1917 Annual Report as School Medical Officer for Bootle provides examples of the rather basic nature of some matters that came up in school inspections. He complains about the 300–400 girls who persistently attended school with their heads in a 'verminous condition', and warns that,

Left:
A Central Council for Health Education lantern slide, 1929

Right:
Punch's view of a School Medical Officer's attempt to test a pert child's eyes in front of her giggling classmates. Wood engraving by F. H. Townsend, 1909

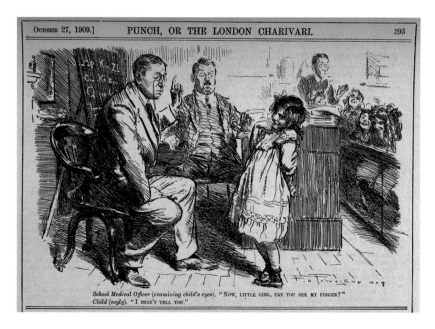

OCTOBER 27, 1909.]   PUNCH, OR THE LONDON CHARIVARI.   293

School Medical Officer (examining child's eyes). "NOW, LITTLE GIRL, CAN YOU SEE MY FINGER?"
Child (coyly). "I SHAN'T TELL YOU."

persuasion and threats having failed, public facilities for voluntary or compulsory cleansing might have to be provided. He draws attention to the absence of pocket handkerchiefs and of toilet paper in the latrines and suggests that class teachers might usefully give some training in personal hygiene. On a more optimistic note, Daley was able to report that the School Canteen Committee had distributed 1,136 pairs of clogs, mainly through the delightfully named 'Clog Clubs' that had been formed to enable children to purchase clogs at less than cost price. Daley, incidentally, had become MOH for Bootle at the age of 24 after his father, who was only 47, had drowned in a yachting accident. He was eventually knighted and made honorary physician to George VI, and his papers are now in the Wellcome Library.[2]

'Slaughter of the innocents'

In the early years of the twentieth century, infant mortality continued to be a matter of concern. In his 1907 annual report John Crome, MOH for Blyth Urban District Council, points out that over a tenth of the children born in that district did not live through their first year, saying, 'this surely is the slaughter of the innocents'. All kinds of remedies had been tried and various incentives offered, such as money prizes for parents of babies who had succeeded in reaching the age of one – which had apparently proved 'eminently successful' in Huddersfield.

The very high death rate among young children was also a problem in the newly created metropolitan borough of Finsbury, a poor and overcrowded area of London with a growing immigrant population, where the MOH was George Newman (who, like Daley, was ultimately knighted and whose papers are also housed in the Wellcome Library[3]). His annual reports are substantial and lengthy – over 250 pages each for 1903 and 1904. He often included special reports on topical issues, such as his 1903 'Special Report on Aliens', which provides a vivid picture of life for the 1,400 or so Italians who were living in Finsbury at the turn of the century.

He lists the Italians' occupations: some made ice-cream, or played the organ; others were asphalters, pavers, mosaic-floor workers, plaster-model makers (with a description of the plaster-

George Newman's graph
showing infant mortality
due to diarrhoea in
relation to fluctuations
in temperature during
1904 in Finsbury, London

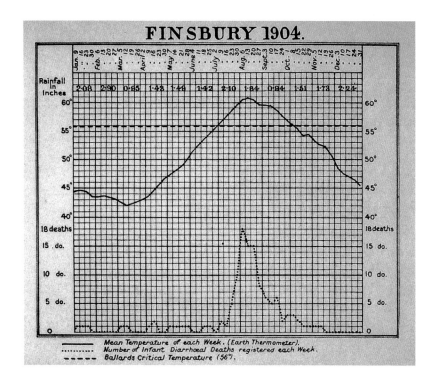

cast process practised by the Italians) and masons. The head
of a well-known asphalting firm which employed thirty to forty
Italians told him that Italian asphalters were preferable to English
workmen for two reasons: they were more reliable and they could
stand the heat of hot new pavements better than Englishmen.
Newman also suggests that the Italians took better care of their
children, who were healthier than their English neighbours: infant
mortality among Italians in London was much lower than among
a similar class of English in the same district. But not everything
the Italians did was perfect: their barrel-organ playing, for example,
was a public nuisance.

Care in the community

The 1940s brought radical changes, as a result of the war and the
introduction of the National Health Service. The contraction in the
social responsibilities and interests of MOsH, with the loss of hospital

and maternity care services to the NHS, proved discouraging to many of them. Infectious diseases were mostly no longer the concern they had been – though polio provided a brief spurt of excitement in the late 1940s and early 1950s and TB eradication measures took up time in the same decades. In the years after 1950, when the overriding emphasis on infant mortality that had marked the early years of the twentieth century had all but disappeared, MOH interests shifted again and care of mentally and physically disabled people and the aged and infirm, almost invisible in the MOH reports at the beginning of the century, emerged as a public health concern.

Society of Medical Officers of Health

In addition to MOH reports, the Wellcome also holds the archives of the Society of Medical Officers of Health, which was founded in 1856 after the passing of the Act which divided London into Metropolitan Districts and required each to appoint an MOH. The Society was based in London, but from 1859 it allowed MOsH from outside the capital to join.[4]

The collection provides a well-documented history of the Society's origins, development and decline, as well as of public health in Britain from the mid-nineteenth century, and includes its official journal, *Public Health*. This was started in 1888 and is an invaluable source of information on all sorts of public health topics from smallpox to Swedish dust carts, sewers to oysters, slum housing to welfare of gypsies, health service management to the teaching of housewifery, and food regulation to the health of immigrants.

Among the archive's twentieth-century material are pamphlets, booklets, leaflets, reports, regulations, government circulars, journals, articles and newspaper cuttings covering different aspects of public health services and policies, such as health centres, maternal mortality, nutrition, smoke abatement, food regulation, health education and more. A booklet published by the National Smoke Abatement Society around 1950, entitled *Britain's Burning Shame*, features the evil 'Sammy Soot', and shows how a smoky atmosphere generated by industrial pollution can wreck your marriage, ruin your complexion, pollute your food, impair the growth of your children and increase your cost of living. Phew.

PUBLIC HEALTH
RELATED COLLECTIONS

In the early years public health was almost entirely male-dominated, but towards the end of the nineteenth century women began to play more of a part. The very first 'health visitors' had been appointed in 1863 by the Ladies' Sanitary Reform Association of Manchester and Salford, and in 1893 two women sanitary inspectors were appointed in the London Borough of Kensington. But the real breakthrough came in 1878 when, after a long and uphill struggle spearheaded by Sophia Jex-Blake, who founded the London School of Medicine for Women in 1874, the University of London Senate agreed to grant degrees to women in all their faculties. Edith Shove was appointed the first woman Medical Officer to the Post Office in 1883, less than a year after she graduated in medicine at the University of London, one of the first two women to do so. By the early 1900s posts in the field of public health were increasingly open to women, who were being appointed Assistant MOH and School Medical Officer, if not Medical Officer of Health.

Dr (Josephine) Letitia Denny Fairfield (1885–1978)

Letitia Fairfield (the novelist Rebecca West's elder sister) had a distinguished career in public health and became the first woman senior medical officer at the London County Council. When war broke out in 1914 she was one of a group of women doctors who offered their services to the War Office, only to be told that their contribution was not needed. By 1917, however, the shortage of manpower had brought about a change in attitude, and she was appointed a medical officer to the new Women's Army Auxiliary Corps, and then, in June 1918, chief medical officer to the new Women's Royal Air Force. Fairfield returned to work at the LCC in 1920 and was called to the bar in 1923; medico-legal matters were another of her professional interests. During the Second World War she became the senior woman doctor and assistant director-general for medical services, but in 1942 she reached the compulsory retirement age for the army and returned to the LCC, where she continued to work up to the formation of the NHS in July 1948.

Throughout her working life Fairfield was involved in contemporary social controversies. As a medical student and young doctor she played an active part in the campaign for women's suffrage and addressed many public meetings. She joined the Fabian Society in London, spoke in public and wrote regularly on issues of women and health. She was also strongly committed to the cause of Irish independence. Having become a Roman Catholic in 1922, for many years she contributed regularly to the Catholic press on such matters as medical evidence for miracle cures, the supernatural and exorcism.

The Wellcome's collection of Dr Fairfield's papers reflect her interests in social hygiene, in mental health, in medico-legal matters and criminology, mother and child health and welfare, and as a Roman Catholic convert, as well as her broader political and feminist convictions.[5] There are typed transcriptions of interviews and reminiscences and personal and family biographical material, including an angry correspondence about her sister Rebecca's unflattering portrayal of her in Rebecca's thinly disguised work of 'fiction', *Family Memories*.

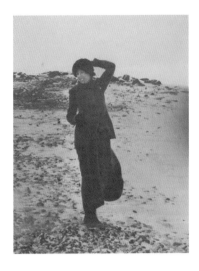

Letitia Fairfield at a pre-First World War Fabian summer school at Barrow House in the Lake District

Dame Janet Maria Vaughan (1899–1993)

The Wellcome Library has a small collection of the papers of Dame Janet Vaughan, haematologist and radiobiologist, mainly covering the years 1939–49, including her work with the Emergency Blood Transfusion Service, social and industrial medicine and postwar medical services, child guidance, the Health Survey and Development Committee in India, and the treatment of sufferers from starvation liberated from Belsen.[6]

The unforgettable experience of the Belsen Camp investigation emerges with shocking clarity in the various reports in the file, produced by Vaughan and her two companions, Rosalind Pitt-Rivers, biochemist, and Charles Enrique Dent, physician and biochemist (some of whose papers are also in the Wellcome[7]). In a typescript of a report Dame Janet presented to the Inter-Allied Conference on Military Medicine, she describes their difficulty in communicating with the Russians, Poles, Yugoslavs and Czechs who formed the majority of the camp inmates. These had come to regard doctors and nurses as people 'who came to torture rather than to heal'. If they were approached with a stomach tube, 'they would curl themselves up and say *"Nicht crematorium"*.' Dame Janet and the others soon understood why – in the camp the custom had been to inject 'moribund' patients with benzene in order to paralyse them before removing them to the crematorium.

… while you have all heard a great deal about the horrors of Belsen, the world has heard far too little of what was done by that handful of English men and women who went in to cope with one of the most immense medical problems that has ever confronted anybody. We arrived a fortnight later, but I think that both I and my colleagues will always feel that it is one of the highest privileges we have ever had to see what courage and kindliness can do in the face of the most tremendous difficulties which most of us would have felt to be almost insurmountable …

From 'Experiences of Belsen Camp', a paper Dr Janet Vaughan presented to the Inter-Allied Conference on Military Medicine, 4 June 1945

The Health Visitors' Association

In 1896, seven women sanitary workers, all based in London, founded the Women Sanitary Inspectors' Association, which expanded into the organisation now known as the Health Visitors' Association, whose extensive archive includes a rich collection of publications.[8]

Its members worked in a variety of settings: homes, schools, workshops, factories, health centres, clinics and hospitals; and the records of the Association cover many social aspects of health and disease. The Wellcome holds an almost complete run of the Association's journal from its first appearance in 1927 under the title *The Woman Health Officer* – which was changed to *Health Visitor* in 1964.

Among the HVA records are small collections of papers belonging to individual health visitors such as G. K. Burne (1912–1989), who worked as a District Nurse in Nevis, Leeward Islands, British West Indies, from 1943 to 1946, and at the Harcourt Health Centre in Hong Kong from 1947 to 1962 as Supervisor and Training Officer of Health Nurses. Burne undertook surveys in Nevis on infant mortality, illegitimacy and paternal care, and there is an intriguing file about the puppetry techniques which she developed for Hong Kong Chinese health visitor trainees to use in health education work. An amateur film she made at the Harcourt Health Centre in 1954, entitled *Students of Mother Craft*, shows mothers, babies and trainee health visitors at an infant welfare clinic in glorious 1950s Technicolor.

Pioneer Health Centre, Peckham (1926–50)

The Pioneer Health Centre was an important experiment in community health. Based on the idea that doctors were treating 'illth' rather than promoting health, the initial aim was to discover what factors achieved the latter. Commonly known as the Peckham Project, it sought to provide regular health check-ups in a community where membership focused on families, rather than individuals. It was the brainchild of George Scott Williamson (1883–1953) and

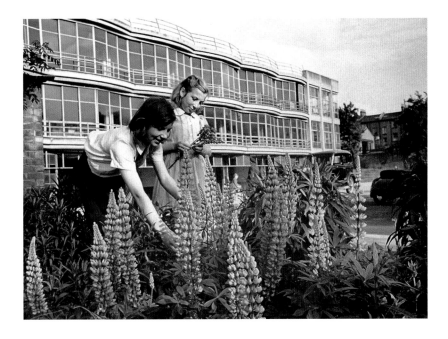
Picking flowers outside the purpose-built Pioneer Health Centre at Peckham, designed by the architect Sir Owen Williams, which opened in 1935

Innes Hope Pearse (1889–1978 – one of the first female medical registrars at the London Hospital), and a substantial part of this collection is made up of their papers.[9]

The centre had to close during the Second World War, when the building was used as a factory for making spare parts for bombers. But it reopened in 1946 and carried on for a few more years before it was forced to close permanently. Finance was always a problem; the membership was never sufficient to enable the Centre to become self-supporting. Insistence that members should pay militated against any absorption into the NHS, and it was at odds with the prevailing models of medical provision. But the Centre has continued to generate both inspiration and controversy. Scott Williamson and Innes Hope Pearse married in 1950, and three years later Scott Williamson died. Innes Hope Pearse lived until the end of 1978.

FORCEFUL AND FORTHRIGHT: W. H. BRADLEY

by Anne Hardy

Among the archive collections that complement the Library's holdings of Medical Officer of Health reports are the papers of James Randall Hutchinson (1880–1955) and William Henry Bradley (1898–1975). These relate to their work at the Ministry of Health from the date of Hutchinson's appointment in 1919, and deal with a wide range of topics from epidemiology through hospitals to vaccination.[1]

Hutchinson and Bradley were both distinguished for their talents as epidemiologists. Hutchinson was said to embody 'the classical tradition of public health epidemiology'. Bradley inherited from him the practice of applying medical science to public health work, which he expounded with infectious enthusiasm, establishing an international reputation in communicable disease control.

Bradley joined the Ministry as a Medical Officer in September 1939. His appointment, like that of many of his predecessors under the Local Government Board, demonstrated an official openness to unconventional career paths. The son of a Post Office engineer, he had joined the Queen's Westminster Rifles on leaving school in 1916. Severely wounded at the battle of Cambrai in November 1917, he became interested in medicine and went on to study at Oxford and Guy's Hospital, qualifying in 1924. He became resident Medical Officer at Downside School (1925–35) and also practised locally as a GP (1930–35).

His observations at Downside triggered his interest in epidemiology and he began to write research papers, notably on respiratory infections. In 1936 he travelled to the United States on a travelling studentship from Guy's Hospital, with assistance from the Rockefeller Foundation. On his return he worked as a research assistant in Cambridge under John Ryle, then Regius Professor of Medicine, who had a profound influence on him.

His reputation as an epidemiologist apart, Bradley's career carried many hallmarks of success. He was promoted to Senior Medical Officer in 1946 and Principal Medical Officer in 1956. He produced 78 publications, not including contributions to reports, reviews and handbooks, and his lively intelligence is evident in many of his writings.

Bradley was a forceful character with forthright views. Though these were tempered by the warmth of his personality (he was greatly loved by his colleagues), they occasionally put him on the wrong side of the rigid codes of the civil service, notably on occasions when he was dealing with the press and publicity surrounding outbreaks of infectious disease. As a result, his election to the Fellowship of the Royal College of Physicians was delayed until he was 70, and his name never appeared on the Honours List. On his retirement from the Ministry in 1963, he was for several years Visiting Professor at the Epidemic Research Unit, Cornell University, New York, before ill health undermined his physical and mental energies.

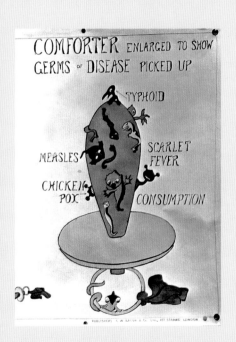

Graphic representation of germs liable to be picked up by a baby's dummy dropped in the street – from the *Daily Mail* Ideal Home Exhibition, 1920

❖

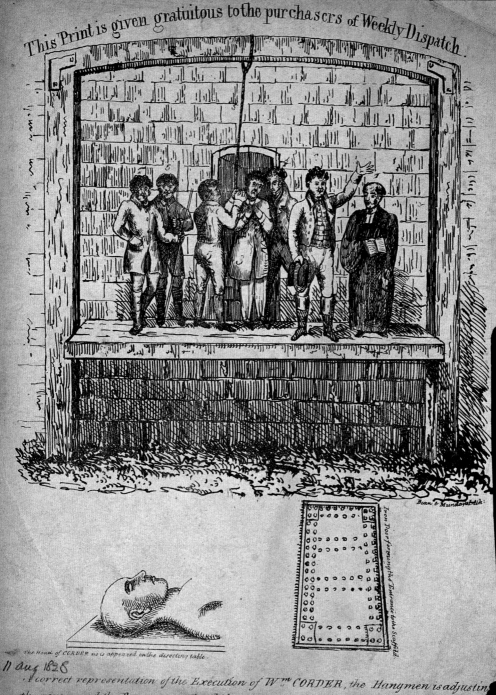

This Print is given gratuitous to the purchasers of Weekly Dispatch.

Bean & Munday, Sc. del[ell?]

Iron Door forming the Entrance to the Scaffold.

The Head of CORDER as it appeared on the dissecting table.

11 Aug 1828

A correct representation of the Execution of W.m CORDER, the Hangmen is adjusting the rope round the Prisoners neck, while an Assistant is supporting the wretched ma[n]

M.r Orridge is announcing CORDER. acknowledgement of the justness of his sentenc[e]

6
WICKED AS EVER: UNTIMELY DEATHS AND EXECUTIONS

No one needs reminding that death comes to us all, but sadly it comes much earlier for some than for others. As a result, tales of suicide, accident, illness, disease, poverty, war, crime and punishment punctuate the Wellcome Library collections. But do not be deterred by these very sobering subjects. Strong stomachs are not a prerequisite for reading further, only an interest in people born into ordinary lives who experienced early, unquiet ends.

The Parish Clerks' Company of London monitored causes of death in the metropolis in their *Bills of Mortality*. These were printed from the 1660s through to the 1830s, and many of them are preserved in the Wellcome's Rare Books Collection. They reveal a great variety of causes of death, many of which would go under the heading of untimely. To take a single example, the week beginning 28 July 1668 saw the following selection of familiar, and less familiar, causes:

Cancer	1
Childbed	4
Convulsions	33
Griping of the guts	84
Measles	2
Rickets	2
Suddenly	1
Teeth	31
Thrush	7

Apart from disease, the *Bills* reported casualties and accidents. In this particular week two suicides were also recorded: 'Hang'd herself at Stepney one, and hang'd himself (being distracted) at Saviours Southwark one.' Only eight people are given 'Aged' as a cause of death during that week.[1]

In the past, bodies had a financial value. Leaving aside the wishes of the dead or their associates, medical schools needed corpses for teaching purposes. Until 1832, however, surgeons were limited by law to using only the bodies of executed murderers for their dissections. Items in the Rare Books Collection indicate how small a number of people this actually amounted to. In the *Bill of Mortality* for the week 27 October to 3 November 1668, for example, just one execution is recorded.[2] In these texts only numbers are preserved, not names. But this particular occasion was immortalised in one of *The Newgate Calendar*'s multi-volume books of criminal stories. There we learn that the condemned man was Thomas Savage, an apprentice who killed a maid. His execution on 28 October was bungled. Having revived after the executioner's first attempt, Savage had to be hanged a second time.

Previous page:
The execution of William Corder, 1828; above, the hangman prepares the noose and, below, Corder's head and shoulders on the dissection table

Right:
The *Bill of Mortality* for the City of London for the week beginning 13 June 1665

The Diseases and Casualties this Week.

Abortive	2
Aged	27
Ague	1
Bedridden	1
Bleeding	1
Childbed	7
Chrisomes	10
Consumption	103
Convulsion	28
Cough	1
Dropsie	24
Drowned at St. Kather. Tower	1
Feaver	48
Flox and Small-pox	8
French-pox	2
Frighted	2
Griping in the Guts	25
Hanged her self at St. James Clerkenwel	1
Jaundies	4
Imposthume	5
Infants	8
Kingsevil	3
Kild two, one with a fall at St. Albans VVoodstreet, and one with a fall from a Scaffold at St. Giles in the fields	2
Lethargy	1
Overlaid	1
Palsie	2
Plague	168
Rickets	15
Rising of the Lights	6
Scowring	4
Scurvy	1
Spotted Feaver	23
Stilborn	9
Stone	3
Stopping of the stomach	5
Strangury	1
Suddenly	2
Surfeit	18
Teeth	19
Thrush	5
Winde	2
Wormes	12

Christned { Males — 101 Females — 103 In all — 204 } Buried { Males — 305 Females — 310 In all — 615 } Plague — 168

Increased in the Burials this Week — 57

Parishes clear of the Plague — 111 Parishes Infected — 19

The Assize of Bread set forth by Order of the Lord Maior and Court of Aldermen, A penny Wheaten Loaf to contain Nine Ounces and a half, and three half-penny White Loaves the like weight.

Murder most foul

Murderers are well represented in the collections, especially medically trained ones. Dr William Palmer, christened by the press 'The Rugeley Poisoner', was convicted of killing John Parsons Cook and executed in 1856 at Stafford. It was commonly believed that the doctor also murdered at least twelve others, including his children, wife and brother, to benefit from their life insurance policies. The sensation this caused is evident in the special Palmer issue of the *Illustrated Times* held by the library.[3] Two of the doctor's letters to his wife can also be consulted, giving a glimpse of just how normal their relationship once had been.[4]

I have been visiting my patients and I must say I feel sick and tired of them.

From an undated letter from William Palmer to his future wife and victim, Annie Brookes

Just over half a century later, Dr Hawley Harvey Crippen was hanged for poisoning his unloved wife, Belle Elmore. Although the poisonous alkaloid Crippen gave her was effective, his mistake was to use slaked lime, instead of quick lime, in an attempt to destroy his wife's body; all that it did was preserve it. Between the poisoning and his apprehension, Crippen carried on working for his employer, The Aural Remedies Company. The library owns a letter he sent to a client during this time.[5] A photograph of Crippen in the dock, taken surreptitiously in court with a Blocknote camera, hidden in a top hat, is another rarity.[6]

Murder was certainly not the only crime that might result in felons breathing their last on the gallows. *An exact list of the several Clippers & Coyners, Highway-men. Foot-padds. House-breakers. Murtherers. And Other Malefactors. which have been executed at Tyburn* gives an indication of the numbers executed in London for murder in the seventeenth century.[7] Far more were executed for burglary and highway robbery than for murder. The deterrent value of this harshest of punishments was questionable. After all, as the compiler of this sheet gloomily notes, 'the Execution is no sooner over, than forgot, and Men grow as Wicked as ever …'

I do assure you there is not a single hour of the whole day passes but what you are uppermost in my thoughts & I do think you'll not forget me when I'm away from you. My dearest I hope you will favour me with a few lines by tomorrow night's post as I'm not able to get over before Tuesday.

From an undated letter from William Palmer to his future wife and victim, Annie Brookes

During many weeks past, public attention to this extraordinary case had been kept alive by daily paragraphs in the papers – now describing Palmer's health – now publishing reports on his pecuniary affairs – now giving details of the extensive preparations being made for the trial. The demand for tickets swelled with every paragraph. It was whispered abroad that fabulous prices had been given for places – till, to the honour of the Old Bailey doorkeepers, and the dismay of the moneyed classes, it was announced that money would not be a passport to the court.

Opening paragraph of article on William Palmer in the *Illustrated Times*, 27 May 1856, p. 1

19.

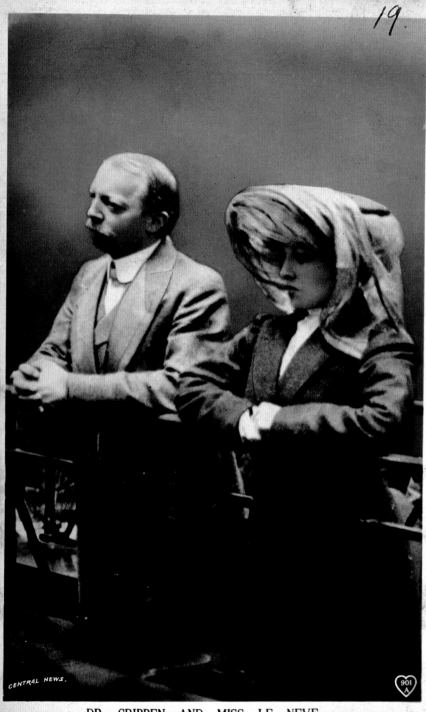

901
A

DR. CRIPPEN AND MISS LE NEVE.

Most strongly do I urge you, therefore, to fill in the enclosed Analytical Form and return it to me without delay, when I will at once send you my opinion on your case. Remember that this costs you nothing at all and places you under no obligation of any kind.

From a letter written by Hawley Harvey Crippen while working for The Aural Remedies Company, 4 April 1910

The London Burkers

Bodysnatchers provided the shortfall in bodies to dissect by digging up the freshly buried and delivering them to the medics. In 1831 John Bishop, Thomas Williams and James May went a fatal step further. Following Edinburgh's William Hare and William Burke's example, these three men caused a sensation when they were found guilty of the murder of a boy they had delivered for dissection. The

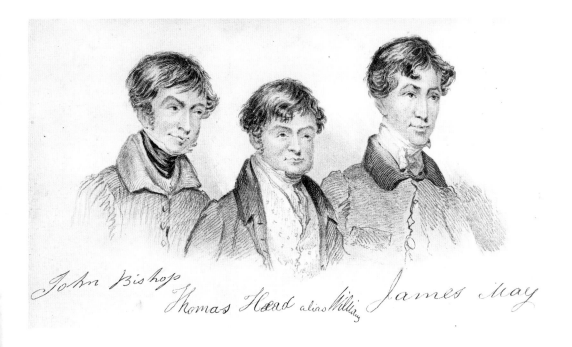

John Bishop Thomas Head alias William James May

Archives and Manuscripts Collection includes a fascinating folder of material on the case of the 'London Burkers' that illuminates the men behind the headlines.[8]

James May's feelings of desperation and anger at the verdict against him are preserved in a little poem he wrote after sentencing. Found in his cell, the slip of paper reads:

James May is doomed to die
And is condemned most innocently
The God above he Knows the same
And will send a mitigation for his Pain.

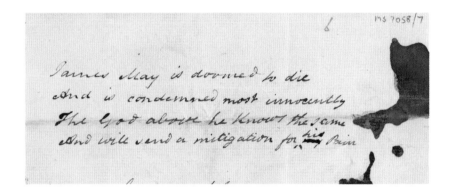

In fact, May never reached the scaffold. His sentence was changed at the last minute to transportation for life, and the papers in the library indicate why. After they were condemned, John Bishop and Thomas Williams made full confessions, witnessed by the Keeper of Newgate Prison. Williams exonerated May from the murder, if not the crime of bodysnatching, declaring in the manuscript: 'The prisoner May was never made acquainted how we came into the possession of the body, or wether the body was murdered or taken from a grave and this is the whole truth I most solemnly declare in the presence of my Maker.'

By declaring May's innocence of the greater crime, Williams helped save his life. But his own life was forfeit. At Newgate two days later, on 5 December 1831, Williams and Bishop were executed in front of a crowd that numbered in the region of 35,000. Their bodies were then dissected, and their remains publicly exhibited.

The Trials

Of John Bishop, Thomas Williams, and James May, for the Horrible

MURDER OF AN ITALIAN BOY

Old Bailey, Dec. 2.

This morning at an early hour the doers of the Court were surrounded by an immense body of people, whose anxiety to witness the trial of the following prisoners surpassed any thing before known.

The Learned Judgs having taken his seat on the Bench, and a most respectable jury sworn,

John Bishop, Thomas Williams, & James May were put to the bar, on the charge of having, on or about the 3d of November last murdered one Carlo Ferrari, an Italian boy.

The following is the substance of the evidence given on the occasion.

John Davis, a porter at Guy's Hospital, stated thut May and Bishop came there on the evening of Friday the 4th November, bringing a body in a sack, which witness believed to be a young boy or girl, from the leg which he saw protruding through a hole in the sack. He declined buying it, because it was not wanted.

W. Hill, porter at the dissecting room King's College, proved the fact of the body having been brought there on the Saturday, as he had described in his evidence before the magistratc. He was sure the body could never have been laid out or buried, and there was blood about the mouth and heart, which appeared to have been wiped off.

Mr. Beaman, surgeon, deposed, that on Saturday, the 5th inst. he was desired to inspect the body. His death had been caused by violence from blows at the back of the neck, with an instrument like that produced.

Mr. Thomas Mills, dentist, deposed that May called at his house at Newington, and offered him a set of teeth for a guinea ; he remarked that one of the teeth was chipped and did not belong to the set. May replied, " upon my soul to God they all belonged to one head not long since, ann the body from which they had been taken had not been buried at the time." The teeth had portions of the gums rdhering to them, and he gave 12s. for them.

Higgins, the policeman, deposen as to the finding an iron instrument, such as is used by resurrection men, and a brad awl on which were stains of blood. He also stated that the clothes produced were the same which he found buried in Bishop's garden, namely, a small blue jacket, a pair of small trowsers, and a boy's shirt which was torn, and had the button holes bursted ; also anoiher boy's jacket, pair of grey trowsers, and a buff striped toilenette waistcoat.

Margaret King swore that the jacket was exactly like that worn by the Italirn boy, who sue saw at the corner of Nova Scotia Gardens.

Augustin Bruin identified the body.

The learned Judge summed up the evidence, and the Jury found a verdict of Guilty egainst Bishop Williams, and May.

Printed by J. Catnach, Monmouth Ct.

At least they kept their skins. In contrast, the surgeon who dissected the murderer William Corder in 1828 preserved his subject's scalp and bound a book with some remaining skin. It might seem fortunate that the library holds only printed material on the subject. A lithograph given to readers of the *Weekly Dispatch*, depicting the gallows scene and Corder's head on the dissection table, is perhaps enough on this occasion.[9]

Incidentally, there is a fine example of a book bound in human skin in the Wellcome.[10] This was published in Amsterdam in 1663 and contains a series of gynaecological essays by various hands, beginning with a treatise on virginity by Séverin Pineau. Dr Ludovic Bouland, who practised in Paris in the late nineteenth century, had it bound in a piece of skin from a woman who had died in hospital (which he had obtained when he was a medical student in Metz) because such a curious little book – he claimed – deserved a binding in keeping with its subject matter.

Broadsides

Only a handful of people at the time would have seen the London Burkers' original confessions. Many thousands more would have read the printed material generated by the trial and execution. Aside from the copious newspaper coverage, the cheapest and quickest accounts to produce would have been the single-sheet publications, printed on one side only, known as broadsides. These reported the trial's progress.

Broadsides were printed for all hangings across Britain, whether they were high-profile like the London Burkers or more commonplace cases. Due to the ephemeral nature of these sheets, however, only a small proportion of the many millions that were printed now survive. Nevertheless, the library holds a growing collection of them in acknowledgement of their historical value. One is an early nineteenth-century broadside recording the execution at Newgate of two robbers, James Frampton and Andrew Barton.[11] Although their tale does not rate an entry in *The Newgate Calendar*, the literature of the streets remembers them, as does the Wellcome Library.

UNTIMELY DEATHS
RELATED COLLECTIONS
Royal Humane Society

The library holds a variety of manuscript and printed material throughout its collections relating to the Royal Humane Society, founded by two doctors in 1774 'for the recovery of persons apparently drowned'. William Hawes and Thomas Cogan believed the rivers and lakes within London were claiming lives unnecessarily through the widespread ignorance of accident and emergency medicine. The Society's objective was to promote the use of resuscitation, a controversial medical technique at the time. The group sought to disseminate information about resuscitation and encourage its adoption. Monetary awards were given to those who attempted to recover the apparently drowned. The Society's annual reports include details of the lives it helped save. These cases give a fascinating glimpse into London's accident-prone and suicides. On 10 March 1775, Frances Pickup, for example, tried to drown herself in the Serpentine due to the 'embarrassed situation of her husband's affairs, being in hourly expectation of an arrest'.[12]

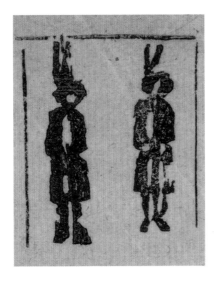

Detail from an early nineteenth-century broadside depicting the execution of two robbers, James Frampton and Andrew Barton

A SERPENTINE TALE

by Ruth Richardson

I've passed much of my adult life in libraries and archives, digging away among all sorts of historical materials. And many of my happiest working days have been spent in Mr Wellcome's great Library.

I'm a nineteenth-century historian, and though I occasionally stray into the eighteenth century, it's rare for me to go back any further than the Georgians. My work has centred on the history of corpse procurement for anatomy, focusing on the 1832 Anatomy Act and its long-term effect, which was to transfer what was widely regarded as a fearful posthumous punishment – dissection – from hanged murderers to the very poor.

At the time of the recent hospital scandal over organ retention, parents whose children's bodies had been ransacked for body parts without their knowledge or consent approached me for help. One had read a book of mine. At first I was uncertain how to respond, but as I saw their situation and how I might assist, I closed my old books for a while and engaged with the present day. I soon found myself invited to speak about the historical context of bodily theft and about what might be learned from the past.

One day, I was feeling particularly overwhelmed with the sense of violation these parents had experienced when they discovered what had been done to their children. Just listening to their stories was harrowing enough. So when I made my way to the library, I may have been seeking a respite.

When I'm researching I often have the feeling there's a guardian angel nearby, alerting me to things I need to find or things I might otherwise overlook. On this particular day, quite unaccountably, I turned up a report of a post-mortem which had taken place in London in 1639.

The description of the pathology was extremely curious, because the surgeon had discovered what he thought was a serpent coiled in the young man's heart. The grieving mother was asked if the surgeon might remove this creature and keep it, but she declined to allow that, saying: 'As it came with him, so it shall goe with him.'

The 'serpent' was probably clotted plasma from the young man's own blood, so his mother's sense that it belonged with him was somehow fitting. But what was most telling for me was that the document provided clear evidence that, although public and professional notions of what properly belongs to the dead may differ, a post-mortem was commissioned and witnessed by an early seventeenth-century London family, and the medical men recognised the family's prior rights to the pathology.

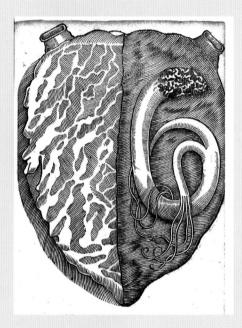

Engraving showing a 'worme' in the right side of the heart, 1639

The discovery enabled me to formulate the view that while understanding human illness may be a joint enterprise, in times of bereavement doctors must learn to accept relatives' limited forbearance of their activities and appetites.

This document, which was so far outside my usual era, was yet so apposite to the turmoil I was experiencing over the unauthorised removal of the children's organs that I felt a guardian angel must indeed have been hovering over me in Mr Wellcome's Library that day.

❖

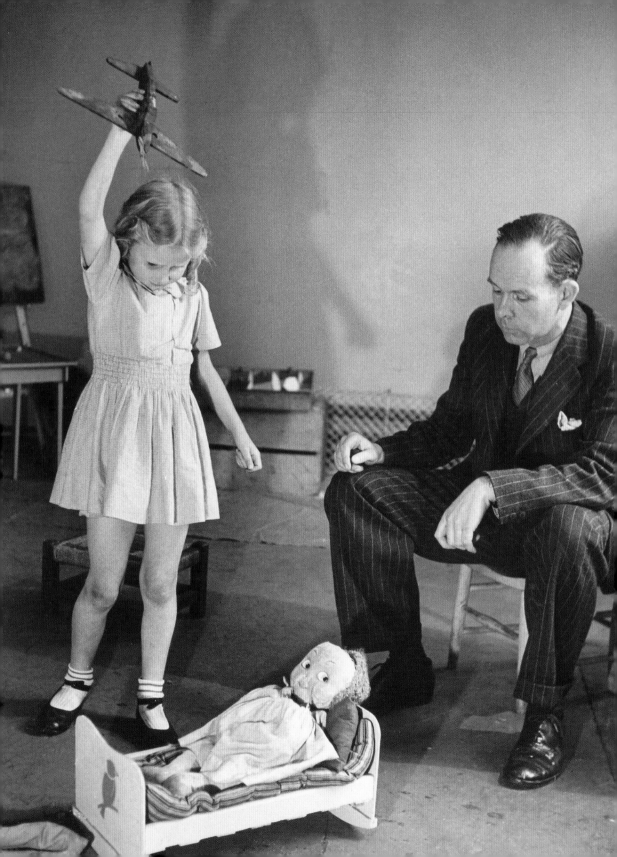

7
MINISTERING TO MINDS DISEASED: PSYCHIATRISTS AND ASYLUMS

Mental disorders have concerned humanity for centuries. There have been numerous ideas about their origins, whether they are treatable and, if so, by what means. The Wellcome Library collections reflect differences of approach over 200 years or so. We can discern an increasing belief that these were not just about control and safe custody (asylum), but that the insane should come under medical management, since the relief, if not cure, of mental distress might be possible. In addition, the notion that there were forms of mental distress that fell outside the parameters of the certification requirements of evolving lunacy legislation was recognised by the growth of the specialism of the 'alienist' during the nineteenth century. With the dawn of the twentieth century, attention turned both to the possibility of early intervention in mental cases, and to questions of preventative strategies of mental hygiene, including the inculcation of mental health in the population at large. Among the most influential movements in understanding the problems of mental functioning and in providing means of alleviation were those related to psychoanalysis.

W hile the Wellcome does not hold the papers of public institutions aimed at providing care, and increasingly treatment, for the mentally distressed (which are public records), Archives and Manuscripts does include some significant records of private lunatic asylums. These were being set up from, approximately, the late seventeenth century to provide institutional care on a paying basis. They were not only aimed at the wealthy; the Poor Law system was required to deal with pauper lunatics and frequently did so by boarding them out in dedicated 'mad-houses' under private management.

Initially, these establishments were not necessarily either owned or managed by medical men: several were under the guidance of clergymen, while others were established by commercial entrepreneurs. But by the late eighteenth century the specialism of 'mad-doctor' was emerging and the idea of medical intervention was gaining currency. The profile of this new branch of the profession, as of insanity in general, was heightened by the madness of King George III and its constitutional consequences. In 1774 came the first legislative attempt to regulate institutions offering care of the insane, by providing for visits and inspection by designated Commissioners, a system which became more regularised and centralised during the nineteenth century.

Names of Patients Under Restraint …
1853 Sept 5 Mr G— hands at night and
Mr O — hands at night, for the same reason as
Mr G —, viz self-abuse. His father requests that
mechanical restraint may be placed upon him.

Ticehurst Medical Journal and Weekly Report, 1845–53

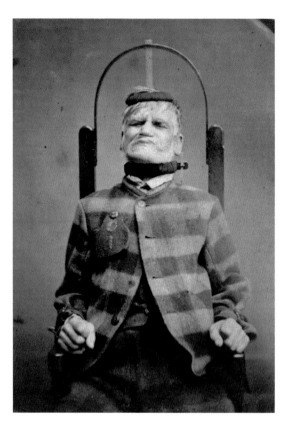

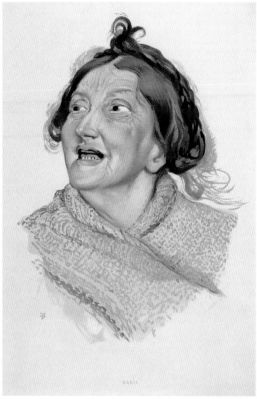

Left:
The photograph of a man clamped in a restraint chair in the West Riding Lunatic Asylum, Yorkshire, c.1869, is attributed to Henry Clarke

Right:
The colour lithograph of 1892 represents a woman diagnosed as suffering from 'hilarious mania'

The largest collection of records of a private psychiatric institution at the Wellcome is that of Ticehurst House Asylum.[1] This was established by Samuel Newington, a qualified surgeon and apothecary, in Sussex in 1792, as a family business – its management remained in the hands of the Newington family for several generations. Though the vast majority of its inmates were private paying patients, and the promotional literature issued by the Newingtons indicates they were aiming at that kind of constituency, a number of pauper patients were also received there during the earlier years. But with the extensive development of public asylums, and the success of the Newingtons in attracting a clientele of a higher class, these admissions dwindled until they ceased during the 1820s. Ticehurst came to receive some very elite patients over the course of the nineteenth and early twentieth centuries, including the 11th Duke of St Albans and the Egyptian Prince Ahmed Saaf Ed Deen.

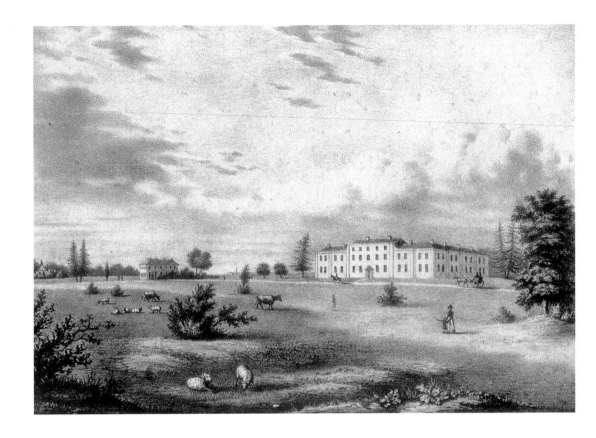

The copious documentation gives a good idea of the elegant facilities: the house which could have been a country mansion set in rolling grounds with a vineyard; the various entertainments and pastimes available to the inmates; the nature of the accommodation. The case records provide substantial information about the patients and their problems, giving a detailed insight into the diagnoses applied, the issues that specially concerned the doctors (such as masturbation) and the various methods of management in practice. The staff/patient ratio was very generous, and the more extreme forms of physical restraint seldom had to be resorted to, though there was also a policy of refusing or transferring patients who were excessively violent.

Ticehurst House private asylum for the insane, from the prospectus of 1827

He is now cleanly in his habits as regards the calls of nature – His attendant informs me that he appears to have 'quite given over his "nasty habit"' – The confinement is still continued – Mr O—— had two tepid baths during the week since Nov 1st – he appears to like them much.

Ticehurst casebooks, 5 September 1853

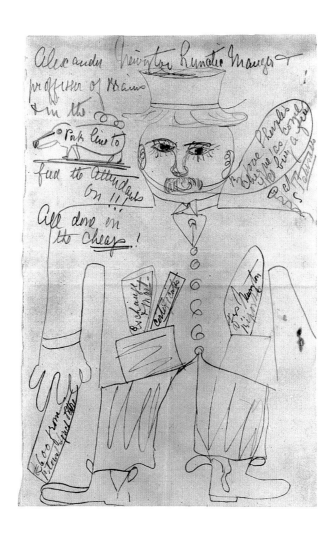

Drawing from 1891 of
Dr Alexander Newington
by a Ticehurst House patient

June 4th. 89 Is still in an acutely maniacal state, incessantly chattering all day — is taking warm baths daily with cold to the head for half an hour at a time — food ordered to be administered every 2 hours — night draughts occasionally.

June 10th 89. Though still maniacal, is much quieter. today she took up a book for about 20 minutes, & looked quietly at the pictures, takes her food well, but sleeps badly — The Baths are still continued

R. Pot Brom 9ᵢᵢ
Tr. Hyos 3i; tᵈˢ
aq 3i; tᵈˢ

June 18th. No change to be reported — She shews a strong aversion

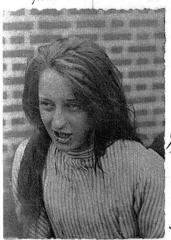

to baths of any kind especially shower baths — though they certainly diminish the excitement at least temporarily — Her appetite is excellent — and she looks considerably better than on admission — The annexed photos. were taken today —

June 25. She remains wild & excited chattering incoherently, jumping, clapping her hands &c — her physical strength is unimpaired —

July. 10. No improvement to be reported.

Aug 10. She is not so noisy & incoherent. but she still walks quickly up & down the airing, attitudinizing, sometimes muttering to herself, at others talking audibly —
she eats & sleeps well —

Sept. 10. Though thinner she is still well nourished — appended is a photograph taken today — Mentally she is quiet & rational though very depressed, at times crying bitterly she thinks her brother is dead — she is now sleeping in a usual general dormitory

From the case notes
of a female patient
at the Holloway
Sanatorium, 1889

Other private asylums had a less exclusive clientele. Camberwell House Asylum in south London (for which two volumes of detailed case records of patients admitted between 1847 and 1853 are held[2]), accepted predominantly pauper patients on behalf of Poor Law authorities from many areas of England which either did not have their own asylums or found Camberwell's rates more economical. The Holloway Sanatorium, however, was specifically intended for 'the Insane of the Upper and Middle Classes'.[3] It was established in the later decades of the nineteenth century following the extensive building of asylums for the poor and represented a new departure, also reflected in the records of Manor House Asylum Chiswick and The Priory, in admitting voluntary 'Boarders' who had not been certified but who (or whose families and friends) thought they would benefit from a sojourn in the Sanatorium. The presence of female doctors on the staff was a further innovation; so too was the inclusion of photographs in the case reports.

He threatened to cut his wife's throat, he thinks that people come into the house to murder him – He chased an imaginary woman out of the coal-cellar into the street & pursued her with a poker – He took his wife for a waiter & offered to pay her – He is exceedingly violent and dangerous.

Holloway Sanatorium Case Book no. 11 Males (admissions 1901)

Aftercare and analysis

Although it is often assumed that, prior to the mid-twentieth century, once an individual was designated as a lunatic and incarcerated in an institution this was a life sentence, the records of nineteenth-century asylums indicate that many of their patients were discharged 'relieved', if not entirely 'recovered', even if there remained a substantial core of long-term inmates. In the 1870s the Reverend Henry Hawkins drew public attention to the problems that might arise with the transition from institutional care to independent living, especially for those members of the community who did not have the support of family or friends on their discharge.

The following are examples of cases assisted:

—A very highly-educated lady, quite destitute, Assisted by gift of clothing, Has obtained a situation as a governess.

—A most respectable girl. Became ill through worry and deprivation in helping her father— a small tradesman who lost his capital. Is now in service in a house of a Member of the Committee.

—A respectable middle aged woman from a Midland County Asylum. After being placed in a Home, obtained work as a dressmaker and is doing very fairly well.

Annual Report of The After-care Association for Poor and Friendless Female Convalescents on Leaving Asylums for the Insane, 1887/88

This led to the inauguration of The After-care Association for Poor and Friendless Female Convalescents on Leaving Asylums for the Insane, which soon extended its remit to men as well. The organisation developed a system of social case-work and established a number of residential homes, either as rehabilitation hostels or providing more long-term sheltered accommodation.[4] It still exists as Together: Working for Wellbeing, since despite enormous medical and social welfare changes the problem it was set up to address remains.

Twentieth-century developments in the treatment of early manifestations of mental illness, as well as in the prevention of psychiatric dysfunctions, were stimulated by the rise of psychoanalysis following on from the work of Freud and his disciples on the continent. A significant figure in the 'British School' was Melanie Klein.[5] Born in Vienna, she came to London in 1926 at the invitation of Ernest Jones and settled there. She is particularly noted for her work with disturbed children, for whom she developed techniques using small toys and analysing their drawings, and for her theoretical insights. Her ideas influenced art critics such as Adrian Stokes. She also analysed adult patients, including several individuals who became influential analysts in their own right. She even analysed her own responses to undergoing a surgical operation, c. 1937.

After Freud came to England with his daughter Anna in the late 1930s, Klein and her adherents increasingly came into conflict with the latter (Anna Freud was also a significant pioneer of child analysis) and her followers. The 'Controversial Discussions' that ensued during the years 1942–3 over practice and training within the British Psychoanalytic Society could be so intense that the participants failed to notice the air-raids going on overhead.

The rise of Nazism during the 1930s led to the arrival in the UK of a number of other significant figures in psychiatry. Sigmund Heinrich Fuchs, who changed his name to Foulkes, arrived in England in 1933.[6] In the Second World War he was involved in the experiments in group therapy taking place at Northfield Military Hospital, and was later a founder member of the Group Analytic Society.[7]

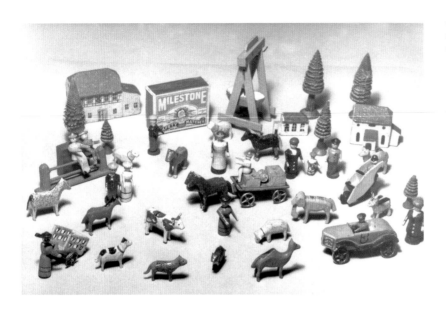

Toys used by Melanie Klein (1882–1960) in her work with disturbed children

[D]eep anxiety situations connected with the inside had, as it were, cut off my relation with external objects. It is, of course, more complicated than this, because I felt very strong gratitude and a very friendly relation to the surgeon, who came to see me every day, and who even seemed to take great interest in some of the psychological aspects which I discussed with him, and who said, quite spontaneously and before I gave him such details, that he feels sure that extremely early fears are stirred by an operation; that it takes one back into quite early times, and that in his view, to recover from an operation is more determined by mastering it psychologically than physically.

Melanie Klein: 'Observations after an Operation', c. 1937

John Bowlby was one of Klein's analysands – though he would come to have differences of opinion with her as his own ideas evolved. In the 1930s he worked extensively in the area of delinquency and child guidance. During the Second World War he served in the Royal Army Medical Corps and played a particularly important role in improving the effectiveness of Selection Boards, mainly for officers. After the war, as a result of work he had done on evacuation, and his study under the aegis of the World Health Organisation of children orphaned or abandoned and institutionalised as a result of war, he developed influential ideas on child development and the role of attachment to the mother or other primary carer. These had a significant impact on policy: for example, it is no longer considered perfectly all right for small children in hospital to be denied parental visiting in case it 'upsets' them. His copious papers also reflect his wide-ranging international connections and shed light on a number of institutions and societies in which he was active.[8]

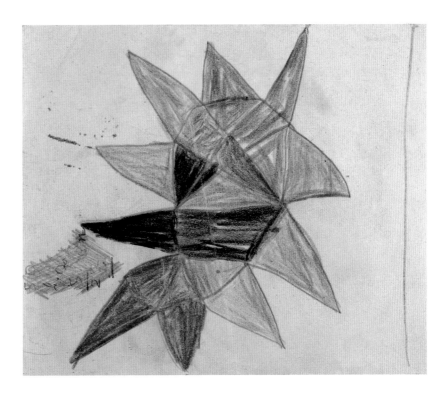

A child's drawing, from Melanie Klein's papers

PSYCHIATRY RELATED COLLECTIONS

Rudolph Karl Freudenberg had been working predominantly with the physical treatments that were finding favour in the 1930s, such as insulin coma therapy, when he came to England with his wife Gerda (also a psychiatrist) in 1937. However, as Medical Superintendent of Netherne Hospital, a large NHS mental hospital in Surrey, during the 1950s and 1960s, he developed an eclectic range of approaches, including art therapy. Freudenberg was also active in the de-institutionalisation that new developments in psychotropic drugs made possible.[9] A more stringent line on the potential of

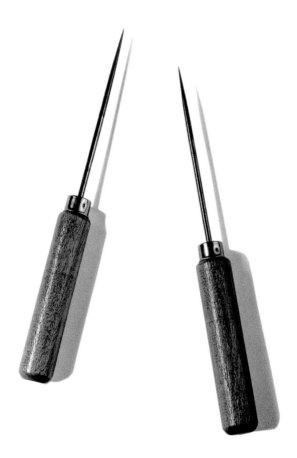

The tools of psychosurgery: a set of Watts-Freeman lobotomy instruments, c. 1950

physical treatments was taken by Dr William Sargent.[10] He was a strong advocate of the use of drug therapies in cases of mental disorder, also electric shock treatment and psychosurgery. His interests included religious and other conversion experiences and the allied area of brainwashing and the phenomenon of false confessions, as well as the legal concept of sanity. The papers of Carlos Paton Blacker include material about his work at the Maudsley Hospital and his involvement in policy-making – for example, working with the Board of Control on keeping appropriate records and generating valid statistics.[11]

Testimony from people suffering from mental distress and disturbance tends to be rare: cases are usually reported by medical attendants rather than recorded directly. But there are exceptions, such as the letters written by Nora Quin to her sister Cissie during her incarceration in the York City Mental Hospital.[12]

Dear Cis
Come and fetch me at once – I cannot
stand this place another day, as a matter
of fact I shouldn't be in it at all.
Don't be so stupid – no so-called Committee
or Mental Doctor in England can keep
a person in a hell-hole like this from morn
till night against their will.

Letter from Nora Quin in the York City Mental Hospital to her sister, c. 1938

These are but a handful of the substantial holdings of Archives and Manuscripts relating to psychiatry – not to mention the monographs, textbooks, journals and annual reports of individual institutions held among the General Collections, or the iconographic and audio-visual material. Two sources leaflets (available online) – *Psychiatry, Psychology, Psychoanalysis: (1) Personal papers*, and *(2) Institutions* – provide an overview of relevant manuscripts and archival collections from the early modern period to the late twentieth century.

Kept under water 5 minutes.
& some seconds not
computed.

Hiurus
Tropidon
gemconates? (Rath-crater

8
BY LAND AND SEA: TRAVELS IN EUROPE AND ASIA

Wherever human beings go, illness and injury follow; and close on their heels come the medical men and women. Diaries, published accounts, scrapbooks and albums kept by practitioners of medicine abound in the Wellcome Library collections. Some document travels in pursuit of a medical vocation; others record holiday travels (in which, however, the writer's eye is usually drawn to matters of health and medicine). Most corners of the globe are covered, often in vivid detail.

Two contrasting documents, both dating from the early nineteenth century, illustrate the genre. In one, the microscopist Joseph Jackson Lister, then in his early thirties, records his journey in 1817 through France to the Alps and home down the Rhine.[1] In the other, an anonymous ship's surgeon, apparently an Irishman, records his passage out to India and back as surgeon of the East India Company ship *William Miles* two years later.[2]

Lister was one of the British tourists who flooded into France after the Napoleonic Wars in the same way that Westerners flooded into Prague after the fall of the Iron Curtain, making journeys that had been difficult to undertake for a generation. At the front of the journal he notes down some travel tips, intended no doubt to instruct the inexperienced: one should always, for example, have written confirmation of the nightly rate you agree with your hotel. Once over the Channel, his journal records all aspects of his travels, from the broad sweep of landscapes and townscapes down to such particulars as the kind of the soil beside the road, peasant costumes and the design of carriages. Bringing a microscopist's eye to the

Previous page:
Watercolour of a snake, from the notebook of the P&O Company surgeon John Temperley Gray, c.1870

Below:
Street scene in Rouen, as recorded on 21 July 1817 by the microscopist Joseph Jackson Lister, father of the more famous Joseph Lister whose pioneering work on antisepsis was a nineteenth-century medical breakthrough, pre-dating the bacteriological revolution

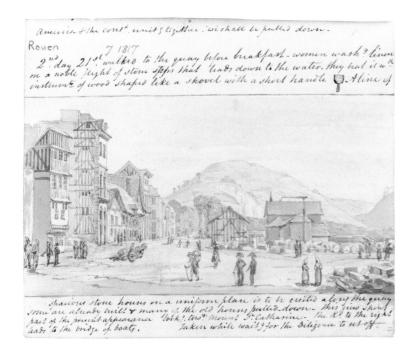

journal, he illustrates the book with exquisitely detailed little pencil or watercolour sketches.

Lister is no sailor: his crossing from Dover to Calais is swift, with the wind dead astern and no need to tack, but he still notes that 'the little vessel was thronged with passengers who were almost all very sick & I for one – lying flat on the back or side I found the best position.' It is a relief when the ship has tied up alongside the long wooden pier at Calais and – 'once my *sac de main* had been searched & I had been stroked down without ceremony by the officers of the Douane' – Lister finds himself ashore. He does not speak French, and as a result has difficulty with the bureaucratic formalities: presenting his passport proves tricky and to reclaim his trunk he retains the services of 'a sharp boy' to be his interpreter and guide.

The surgeon of the *William Miles*, in contrast, is more blasé about the sea: he has certainly made at least one voyage to the Southern Hemisphere before he joins the ship in May 1819. There is drama from the start: he begins his journal, like Lister, in London, but instead of taking the coach to Dover, he boards a small boat and shoots the rapids between the pillars of the old London Bridge:

> … in setting out [I] was fortunate enough to pass through London Bridge at low water when there was nearly 5 feet descent under one of the side arches thro' which we passed. The boat was carried thro' with great velocity but we shipped no sea.

Once at Gravesend, just as Lister did, he makes use of the floating population who made a living hanging about the port to help travellers, for a fee, and his shock at the size of the fee indicates that this may be his first voyage out of London: 'the boatmen truly deserved the name of sharks. They asked [a colleague] & I six shillings for carrying out to the *William Miles* & into shore; gave them 3.' The ship will be his home for the next year; it is, he notes, 'elegantly fitted up', but of course the need to carry food for a long voyage means that 'a most plentifull live stock laid in, 3 cows and a calf – 60 sheep, 50 hogs, 80 dozen of poultry etc. etc which make a most delightful concert in the morning.'

Leisure and self-improvement

The two men pass their days in contrasting fashion. Lister travels southwards in the notorious *diligences* whose discomfort is a constant cause of complaint in travel diaries of the time. He stops frequently, however, seeing the sights of Dieppe and Rouen before his arrival in Paris.

> *We entered Paris by the avenue of Neuilly passing a begun triumphal arch of which only the sides are erected ... On the boulevards in the evening, women who are in want but ashamed to express their distress sing veiled ...*
>
> Joseph Jackson Lister in Paris, 1817

The surgeon of the *William Miles*, on the other hand, leads a more tranquil existence. A recurring feature of shipboard diaries is that the medical man often passes many days without having to practise medicine at all, leaving him free to observe the natural world, learn a language, read up on geology or do whatever takes his fancy. The notebook of John Temperley Gray, a P&O company surgeon who made the same voyage many times later in the nineteenth century, is packed with self-education, drawings of tropical animals or the hats worn by the Parsees of Bombay, and even a musical transcription of a song sung by the men on the docks in India.[3] Similarly, on his two voyages to the Far East in the 1930s, the young Richard Ernest Copithorne treats little but sunburn, a hand crushed in the lifeboat davits and a knife wound picked up by a crewman in Djakarta, and spends most of his professional time organising the ship's library, but fills two volumes with detailed observation of the world around him.[4]

On board the *William Miles*, the days pass without incident, the weather growing warmer and the flying fish accompanying the ship growing more numerous, until the time comes to cross the Equator. The seasoned travellers, the surgeon among them, do their best to prey on the ignorance of the greenhorns on board: 'All the old ones played

Watercolour of a house in Zürich by Joseph Jackson Lister, 1817

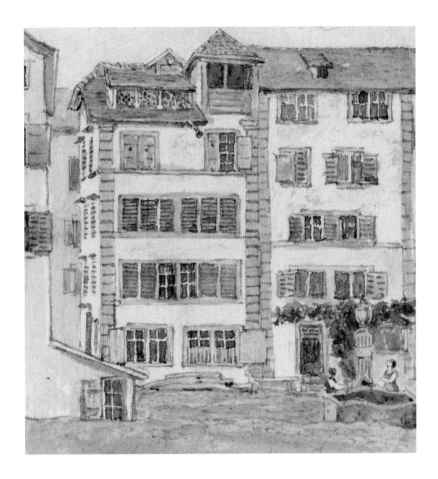

off their tricks… in trying to make the ladies and juniors believe they could see [the Equator]. I did not exactly try so much, but I made them believe me when I told them I thought I could see it.' The following day comes the great ceremony of Crossing the Line.

Lister, too, is travelling further south and further from home. From Paris he makes his way to Switzerland, which – following the fall of Napoleon's Helvetic Republic – was once again a loose aggregation of cantons and city states with their own laws and currencies. Observations of costumes and buildings are superseded by several pages of drawings of landscape (too many, it seems, to finish all of them in watercolour) as he travels up the valley of the Reuss towards the Gotthard Pass. The Alpine tourist explosion was

Neptune's Car (in the shape of a blazing tar barrel) was thrown overboard last evening at dusk, and had a very fine effect ... When the procession was over, the Chief Judge came to the gang way and read out the names of those who had not before obeyed Neptune – and one by one they came up and were delivered over to one of the attendants to be blindfolded – after that they were placed upon a chair and the barber got his lathering brush (a mop) and dipping it into a bucket of a delightful mixture of pitch, grease & other highly odoriferous materials, bedaubed the poor fellow's whole face most plenteously; then taking his razor made of a barrel iron hoop, scraped it all off very carefully not sparing the foundation on which it lay ... This operation was repeated nearly a dozen times, but only on the common men – for the Captain had previously given orders, that the passengers should not be shaved. When the shaving was over the Captain came out and ordering a bucket stood at one of the ports and belaboured us all with water, as long as he could stand ... The ladies seemed to enjoy the fun very much.

William Miles surgeon on Crossing the Line, 1 July 1819

just beginning – two years before Lister visited, hotels had been opened on the Rigi, and in the year before his visit the Graubünden legislature approved a road over the San Bernardino Pass that was to take pressure off the Gotthard, but this was still wild and remote country, and it must have been with relief that he turned north to arrive in Zürich.

The surgeon of the *William Miles*, after a six months' passage, also arrives at the first city for a long time when the ship is anchored in the Madras Roads. For the ship's passengers, however, this is not a return to familiar things but a jarring culture shock: the surgeon relates with amusement how the ladies on deck were startled by the arrival of scantily-clad fishermen; they shrieked and ran below but, he notes sardonically, they soon got used to the sight and were to be seen clustered unconcerned along the rail, gazing upon the new land.

Ashore was a new life with new problems and new excitements for many of the passengers. Household notes recorded at this time by a Mrs Turnbull include recipes for chutneys and curries adapted to British tastes, as well as such useful tips as the need for a preservative to protect wooden furniture from termites.[5]

The return journey

Neither traveller returns by the same route as he took going out. Lister travels north along the Rhine, sketching castles as he goes, and passes through Holland, while for the surgeon of the *William Miles*, the return journey is enlivened when, during the passage of the South Atlantic, the ship puts in at St Helena. There he eagerly collects news about the man who had dominated the past twenty years. Napoleon, apparently, is 'in perfect health, employing himself all day in his garden – dressed in a Nankeen jacket & trowsers – building fortifications to screen him from Observers, into which he runs, like a Rabbit, when he sees anyone approach. He hands the sods himself to the Chinamen about him.'

Both men return to London; Lister after several months and the surgeon of the *William Miles* after a year. Lister returns to his wine merchant's business, his scientific interests and his domestic concerns (he was to be married the following year). His journal forms part of

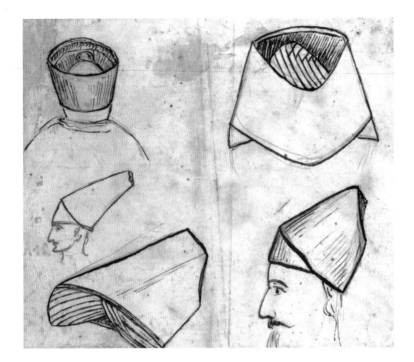

From the notebook of John Temperley Gray: left, sketches of Parsee hats, made in 1862; and below, watercolour of a caterpillar encountered on 11 November 1870

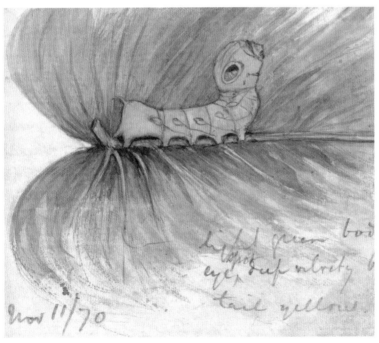

the archives of the Lister family, which centre on the life and work of his son the famous surgeon Joseph Lister.[6]

On his return, the surgeon of the *William Miles* sets off on a tour to the Isle of Wight. Passing through the wooded, hilly country around Hindhead he comes across a stone commemorating 'some horrid murders which happened there'. Twenty years later Dickens sent Nicholas Nickleby along the same road and noted the same stone, with characteristic relish: 'They walked upon the rim of the Devil's Punch Bowl, and Smike listened with greedy interest as Nicholas read the inscription upon the stone which, reared upon that wild spot, tells of a foul and treacherous murder committed there by night. The grass on which they stood had once been dyed with gore, and the blood of the murdered man had run down, drop by drop, into the hollow which gives the place its name.'[7] The stone still stands beside the modern A3.

The surgeon of the *William Miles* is not identified, but it seems that his wandering days were now over: the journal hereafter deals with life in London and breaks off early in 1821. For many, a journey of this nature would be something to do once in a lifetime, something that settling down in medical practice would subsequently rule out.

TRAVEL RELATED COLLECTIONS

The journal of a Mr Pigot, naval surgeon (fl. 1758), covers his passage from Bengal to England, via Arabia, Persia and Turkey (where he was nearly tricked into professing Islam before witnesses and thereby becoming a Turkish subject) between November 1757 and February 1759.[8] On 8 April 1758, he recorded in his journal a truly Arabian Night:

> This evening we were entertain'd at the Baron's House by ye Dancing Girls, (that is Meretrices) who strive to excel each other in ye most lascivious postures of ye Bodies; whilst one was dancing in this manner, ye others who sat around her, accompanying her Motions with Songs and Clapping of their Hands, at ye same time

3 or 4 Men Beat on Drums & join'd also with their Voices; In such effeminate & indecent Diversions ye people of Wealth, & Power, thro'out ye Eastern World take a pleasure & it is ye chief Amusement of ye Life.

A hundred years later, Harry Hayter Ramsdale (fl. 1860) kept a diary while travelling on an emigrant ship in which he briefly took over as surgeon – despite the fact that he had never qualified as a doctor – when the drunken ship's surgeon cut his throat while still in the Channel.[9] The replacement doctor, who was taken on board at Plymouth, was hardly an improvement and Ramsdale had to tread warily when he found his services still very much in demand.

Below left:
Two Afghan women photographed by Lillias Hamilton c. 1896

Below right:
An 1885 photograph of Abd or-Rahman, Amir of Afghanistan, whose personal physician Hamilton became

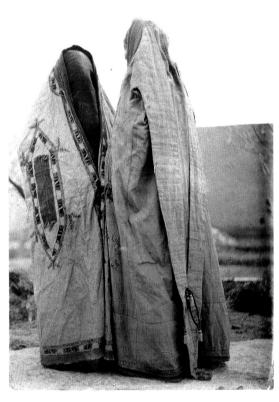

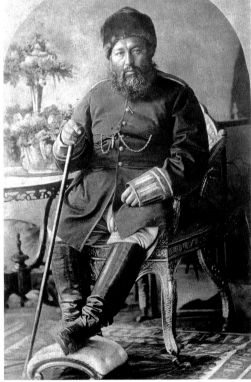

A passport photograph
of Lillias Hamilton
taken in 1920

His diary gives a graphic account of the often petty squabbles that break out when people are cooped up together for long periods on board ship.

The highlight of the life of Lillias Hamilton (1858–1925), whose correspondence and other writings are held in the Wellcome, is probably the period during the 1890s when she became personal physician to the Amir of Afghanistan.[10] She had gone into the hills to recuperate from an illness she had contracted while practising medicine in Calcutta and came to the Amir's attention by curing one of his wives. Hamilton was an accomplished photographer and took many pictures in Afghanistan. Her later life was dogged by ill health, but she still managed to lead an active life as Warden of Studley College in Warwickshire (training women for careers in agriculture and horticulture) for many years, and to serve as a doctor in Serbia during the First World War.

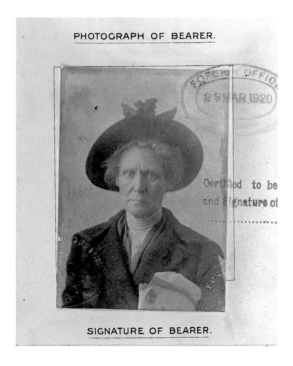

PHOTOGRAPH OF BEARER.

SIGNATURE OF BEARER.

A passport photograph of Lillias Hamilton taken in 1920

YOUNG DOCTORS IN POST-REVOLUTIONARY PARIS

by Gillian Tindall

'I'm afraid the folders don't seem to be in any order ...,' said the librarian in the Poynter Room.

'Then let me have the whole box and I will sort them for you,' I said, and he kindly did.

There is nothing, for a researcher, quite like getting your hands on actual packs of letters, or old-style paper covered in notes for the writer's own eyes, for the past to reach out and touch you. Forget learned articles and definitive biographies, forget (yes, *please*) microfilm or indexes on-line or any other useful modern means of reanimating spent lives: you can't beat original documents that few people have even read, let alone turned into a thesis.

The documents that day were a set of letters written home in 1818 from Paris and various other cities by a young English doctor, plus his own journal which (I presently established) consisted of roughly the same material bulked out with more clinical observation. He was anonymous, but someone had noted that his travelling companion was one John Griscom, a young American whose parallel journal of his year in Europe (which I later ran to earth in the British Library) happened to have been published in New York in 1923. This supplied the name for the doctor; he was John Sims, a physician from Manchester who had just qualified in Edinburgh and was, like Griscom, a Quaker.

Once the bloody dust of the Revolution had settled, Paris benefited from an extraordinary upsurge in scientific thinking. The generation of doctors and surgeons who somehow managed to train in the 1790s proved to be one of the brightest ever, and these were the people whose demonstrations Sims attended. We see in the flesh Dupuytren of the Hôtel-Dieu, performing a rapid operation on a cancer patient 'so as to give the man as little pain as possible'. The red-hot irons were, however, to hand in case of excessive haemorrhage: Griscom began 'breathing hard' and had to be escorted out. Sims also met Dubois, physician to the ex-Empress and guiding spirit of the Parisian midwife-training hospital of which London then had no equivalent, and saw round many other hospitals and asylums whose names still resonate in Paris today. We are with him, with the lunatics at Charenton, in the ex-convents, round the muslin-curtained beds, in

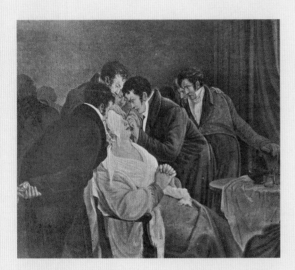

Guillaume Dupuytren of the Hôtel-Dieu operating on a cataract

the dirty dissecting rooms. We visit new Homes for the deaf and dumb and for the blind, and the ancient foundling hospital. We also view the elephant in the Jardin des Plantes and – as another celebrity – the Duc de Rochefoucault, to whom Griscom had an introduction: 'he was standing by the fire finishing a sausage roll, which lay upon the mantelpiece.'

Thank you, John Sims, across 190 years. Thank you, Wellcome Library.

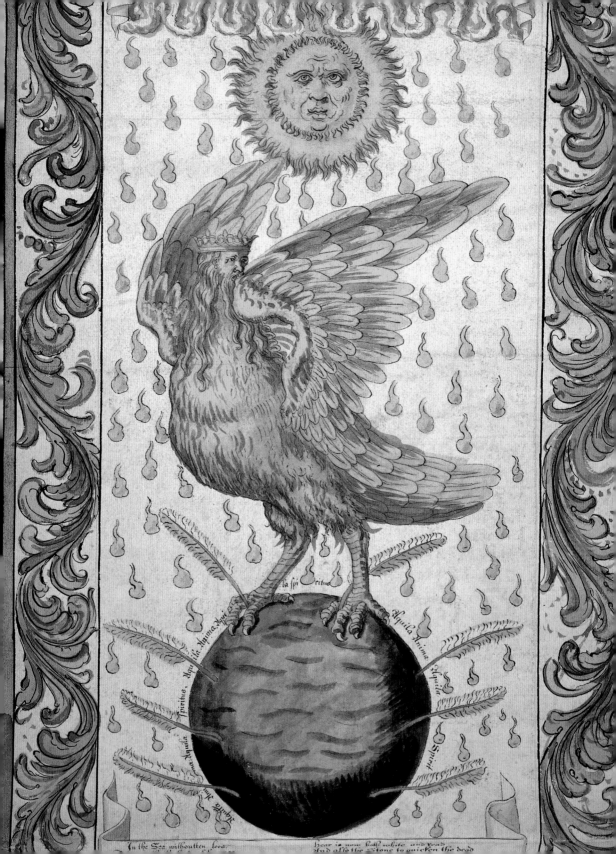

In the See withoutten lees.
hear is now both white and read
And also the Stone to quicken the dead

9
THE ELIXIR OF LIFE: THE MANY FACETS OF ALCHEMY

There is a great deal more to the subject of alchemy than the stereotypical view of the alchemist/magician pursuing the elusive Philosopher's Stone and trying to turn base metals into gold. Alchemy is closely linked to the early history of chemistry and many key figures in the Scientific Revolution, such as Isaac Newton and Robert Boyle, were also serious students of alchemy. There was an important relationship between alchemy and medicine, particularly in the sixteenth and seventeenth centuries with the development of Paracelsianism and chemical medicine (or 'iatrochemistry'). Alchemy also had an essential philosophical basis and developed its own remarkable language of religious metaphor and emblematic symbolism.

The single most important source for alchemical books in the Wellcome Library is the collection of Dr Ernst Darmstaedter (1877–1938). Regrettably the sale of his library proved to be difficult and protracted for both sides, and it ended in tragedy. Darmstaedter was born in Mannheim, studied at the University of Heidelberg, and lived for much of his life in Munich. He wrote extensively on the history of science, specialising particularly in alchemy and early chemistry, and put together a fine collection of early printed books and manuscripts on the subject.

In February 1930 he wrote to L. W. G. Malcolm at the Wellcome Historical Medical Museum saying that he urgently needed to sell the early part of his collection (about 1,500 out of a total of 6,000 items) in order to pay creditors. The books were delivered to London in August 1930, but the sale was not concluded quickly, mainly because of disagreement over books in the original list which had not been handed over. Lawyers were called in by both sides and the final payment was made in April 1931. Darmstaedter continued to have financial problems and, as a Jew, his life in Munich became increasingly difficult. There is further correspondence from him up to 1935, mostly requests for support, academic and financial, to help him publish his research. Sadly, Darmstaedter committed suicide by taking an overdose of barbiturates on 12 November 1938.

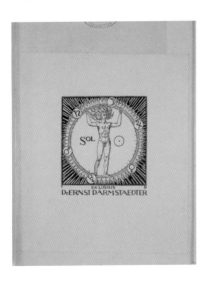

Previous page:
A golden eagle on a sphere, one of the five panels of the 'Ripley Scroll', an alchemical manuscript of the sixteenth century

Left:
The bookplate of
Dr Ernst Darmstaedter

Right:
Jerome Brunschwig's
Liber de arte Distillandi de Compositis,
published in 1512

The Darmstaedter collection contains the most significant works on alchemy and chemistry published in the fifteenth and sixteenth centuries. Amongst these are the first printed edition of the *Summa perfectionis magisterii*, a fourteenth-century text written under the pen name of Geber (Jabir Ibn Haiyan), the eighth-century Islamic alchemist with the same name,[1] the *Liber de arte Distillandi de Compositis* by Jerome Brunschwig, published in 1512,[2] and sixteenth-century editions of Paracelsus, Conrad Gesner and Georg Agricola. One of the scarcest books from the Darmstaedter collection is the *Bericht, vom Bergkwerck*, a treatise on mining written by Georg Löhneyss and published by the author at Zellerfeld in 1617.[3] Many copies were destroyed by a fire during the Thirty Years' War. This copy is in its original stamped pigskin binding with a portrait of Herzog Julius von Braunschweig-Lüneberg, initials I.Z.G.G. and date 1621.

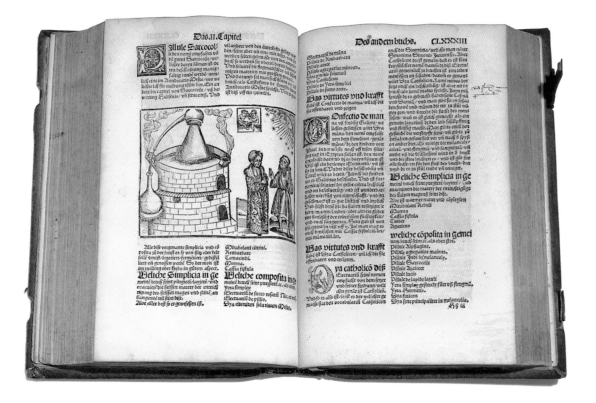

John Dee

There are a number of objects in the collection connected with
the famous astrologer and alchemist John Dee (1527–1608), a true
Renaissance man in the range of his intellectual interests and
practical activities, who is described in Aubrey's *Brief Lives* as
'a mighty good man: a great Peacemaker'. The best-known of these
objects is a crystal, supposedly given to him in November 1582 by
the angel Uriel. Dee, who was Queen Elizabeth I's astrologer, used
the crystal for clairvoyance. In 1640, it was given to the physician,
Nicholas Culpeper (1616–64) by Dee's son, Arthur, as a reward for
curing his liver complaint. Culpeper used it to cure diseases but noted
that its use rendered him weak and liable to be tempted (by a demon)
to acts of lewdness with women and girls. The crystal is now part
of the Wellcome collections at the Science Museum. Hanging in the
Gibbs building, the Wellcome Trust's headquarters at 215 Euston
Road, is a painting by the nineteenth-century artist Henry Gillard
Glindoni depicting John Dee conducting an experiment in the
presence of Queen Elizabeth I and her court.

The 'Ripley Scroll' is one of two alchemical scrolls in the
collection, both over three metres in length.[4] George Ripley was an

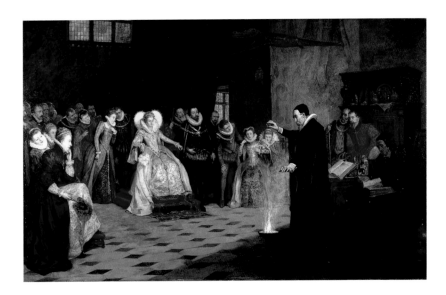

Nineteenth-century
oil painting of John Dee
performing an experiment
in front of Queen
Elizabeth I, by Henry
Gillard Glindoni

Opposite:
Detail from an anonymous
seventeenth-century
manuscript on alchemy

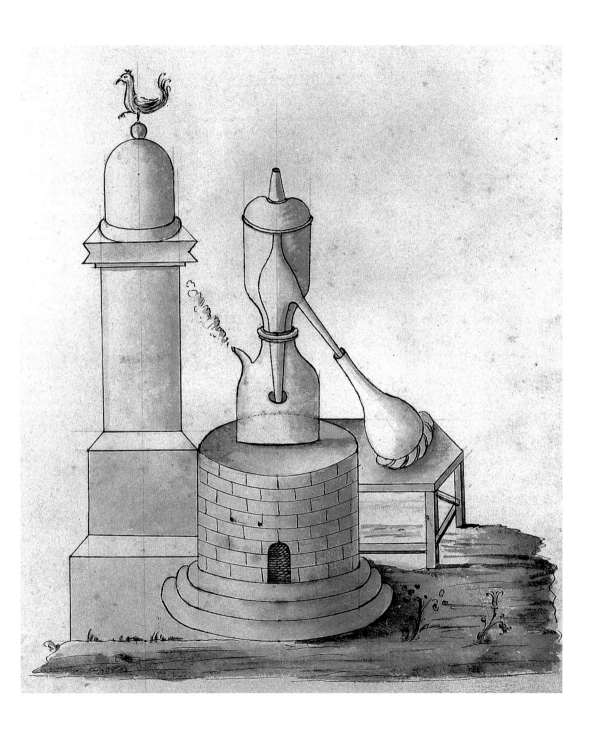

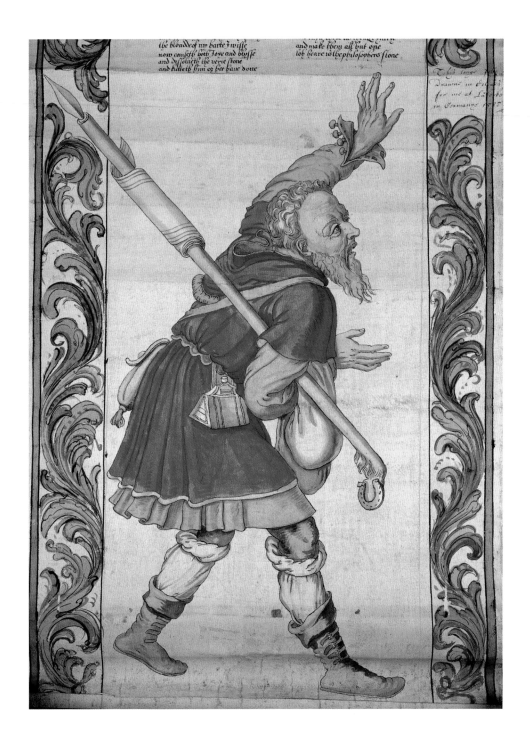

The last panel of the
sixteenth-century
Ripley Scroll, depicting
the 'full-length figure
of the Philosopher'

alchemist and an Augustinian canon at Bridlington in Yorkshire who lived from about 1415 to 1490. He contributed greatly to a revival of the practice of alchemy in fifteenth-century England and his works were copied and republished in the sixteenth and seventeenth centuries. The scroll illustrates the pursuit of the Philosopher's Stone, the vital element in the transmutation of metals and producing the elixir of life. It is divided into five panels: the first is an Alchemist holding an alembic (used in distillation); the next, which is the largest, a fountain supported by a column with many symbolic figures; the third, a golden eagle on a sphere, with the legend 'The Birde of Hermes is my name: eating my winges to make me tame'; the fourth, a large green dragon with other symbols; the last, a full-length figure of the Philosopher, bearing a staff with a scroll wrapped around it, one end being a spearhead and the other a shod horse's hoof. It has been suggested that these were copies commissioned by John Dee.

Also in the collection is an unassuming notebook, wrapped in the printed sheet from a sixteenth-century theological book, which contains alchemical notes written by Dee.[5] It begins with the title 'Practica et accurtaciones Georgii Ryplay et Raimundi' and includes notes on the work of George Ripley and another important mediaeval alchemical author, Raymond Lull. The notes were probably made some time after 1589 when Dee returned to London after spending five years in Poland and Bohemia:

Ther is a body of a body
And a soule and a spirite
With two bodies must be knit

Ther be two earthes as I the tell
And two waters with the[m] to dwell
The one is whit the other red
To quick the bodies that be ded

And one fier in Nature y hidd
And one ayer, w[hich] the[m] doth y dede
And all it cometh out of one kinde
Mark this well man in they mynde

Mary Anne Atwood

An important figure in the nineteenth-century revival of mystical alchemy is Mary Anne South (later Atwood). In 1850 she published, with her father Thomas South, *A Suggestive Enquiry into the Hermetic Mystery*. They immediately decided to withdraw the book and tried to destroy all copies because they believed it was a mistake to reveal the secrets to the world. Consequently copies are now very scarce and the Wellcome copy has a note from Mary presenting it to John Preston and has his emblematic bookplate.[6] Together father and daughter assembled a very extensive library of alchemical works. This was dispersed after Mary's death in 1910 and many items came up for sale at Sotheby's in 1927 in the collection of Walter Travers Scott Elliot. Wellcome bought more than twenty lots at this sale, and several more books were purchased from the bookseller Maggs Brothers the following year. These included one manuscript,

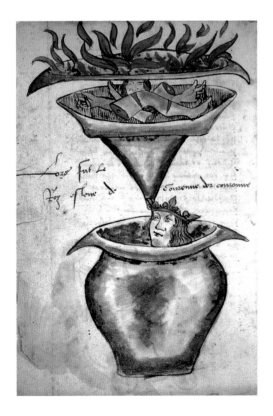

Left:
A detail from Raymond Lull's *Ymage de vie*

Right:
A late fifteenth-century illuminated page from Raymond Lull's book on alchemical processes and receipts

a sixteenth-century collection of alchemical tracts in German.[7] Each of the many important printed books has the bookplate of Thomas South and inscription 'A. T. & M. Atwood 1859' (the year of Mary's marriage to Revd Alban Thomas Atwood).

One of these printed books is a collection of English translations of alchemical works, all published as part of a revival of interest in mystical alchemy in the 1650s, including *The Divine Pymander*, which was attributed to Hermes Trismegistus.[8] The nineteenth-century binding is decorated with emblematic symbols. There is also a copy of *Cabala, speculum artis et naturae, in alchymia* published in Augsburg in 1654.[9] It has the library code of Sir Hans Sloane, one of the foundation collections of the British Museum. It was sold as a duplicate in 1769 and later owned by William Bryan, who has pasted in a mystical manuscript headed 'Wm. Bryan, Born May 4th 1755.M. Given by the Arch-Angel Gabriel July the 1st 1789'.

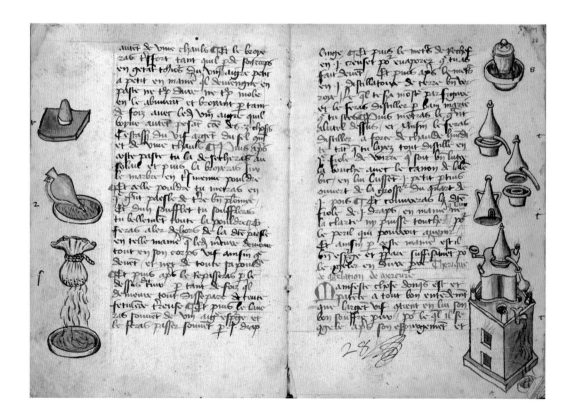

THE MANY MEANINGS
OF MONSTERS

by Armand Leroi

I begin by requesting the Wellcome Library's greatest treasure.
This is Pierre Boaistau's 'Histoires prodigieuses', 1559, a
manuscript presented to Elizabeth I of England by the author
himself.[1] One of the most beautiful of the 'Monster and Marvel'
books of the sixteenth century, it tells of comets that blaze portent-
ously across the sky; a child born with barking canine heads on its
knees and elbows; a pair of conjoined twins who signify a truce
between the warring cities of Genoa and Venice – and much more
besides. It was a pointed gift for a queen, and Elizabeth refused it.
Yet the illustrations are glorious. Another pair of conjoined twins,
this time from Normandy, resembles a pair of Botticelli Venuses
who have become entangled with each other.

I came across this treasure when writing my book *Mutants*. Its
thesis was very simple. Just as developmental geneticists dissect the
molecular pathways that make a worm, a fly or a mouse, so too,
could one dissect a human body. The human genome is vast and
written in an incomprehensible language. Mutations allow us to
translate that language; they are a Rosetta stone for the genome. But
human mutations are different from fly mutations; human
mutations, or rather human mutants, have stories – stories that reach
from the fabulous monsters of antiquity to the biographies of people
whose genes are now the stuff of a thousand papers in the technical
literature of modern genetics.

And the Wellcome Library pullulates with mutants. Like trilo-
bites, one can trace their Modification by Descent. An etching
(English, late eighteenth century) depicts Homer's Cyclops.[2] Of
course, the artist no more believed that Cyclops actually existed than
Turner did when he treated the same theme. Yet some teratologists

argue that Homer's monocular giant was inspired by the congenital deformity that we now know as 'cyclopia'. But in Fortunio Liceti's *De monstrorum* (1634) – arguably the first real teratology (the Wellcome's copy is inscribed by the author to Gussoni) – the Cyclops of antiquity has become a realistically deformed child – albeit one who is an unrealistic three years old, for infants with the disorder are always still-born.[3] Something over a hundred years later, George Leclerc, Comte de Buffon, also illustrates one in his *Histoire naturelle, générale et particulière*.[4] There, along with 'Judith and Hélène, the beautiful Hungarian Conjoined Twins', one finds a cyclopic infant, but dressed in a toga – an allusion to its antique origins.

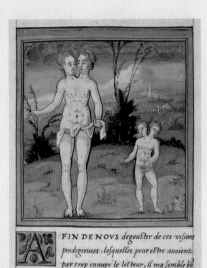

FIN DE NOVS *degouster de ces visions prodigieuses, lesquelles peut estre auoient par trop ennuye le lecteur, il ma semble bõ de.*

A pair of conjoined twins from Pierre Boaistau's 'Histoires prodigieuses', 1559

It is only when I come to the Dutch anatomist, Willem Vrolik, who sought to classify deformed infants as Linnaeus classified beetles – and whose glorious atlas contains pages of cyclopic calves, sheep, cats, fish and humans – that the residue of antiquity is finally stripped away.[5] But even Vrolik subtly falsifies cyclopia, for his lithographs are so beautiful that they anodise the horror of the thing. To bring that home I need Hirst and Piersol's *Human Monstrosities* (1892–3), which, for the first time, has photos of congenital deformities, among them a cyclopic infant, fresh from its formalin, with autopsy sutures running up its abdomen.[6] Finally I go up to the Modern Medicine Room and take down Volume 14 of *Nature Genetics* which contains Roessler *et al*'s classic 1996 paper identifying mutations in the sonic hedgehog gene as the major cause of cyclopia.[7] Portent of divine wrath; senatorial infant; anomalous species; pathology; mutant: the Wellcome Library allows us to choose the meaning of our monsters, but ensures that they are always with us.

❖

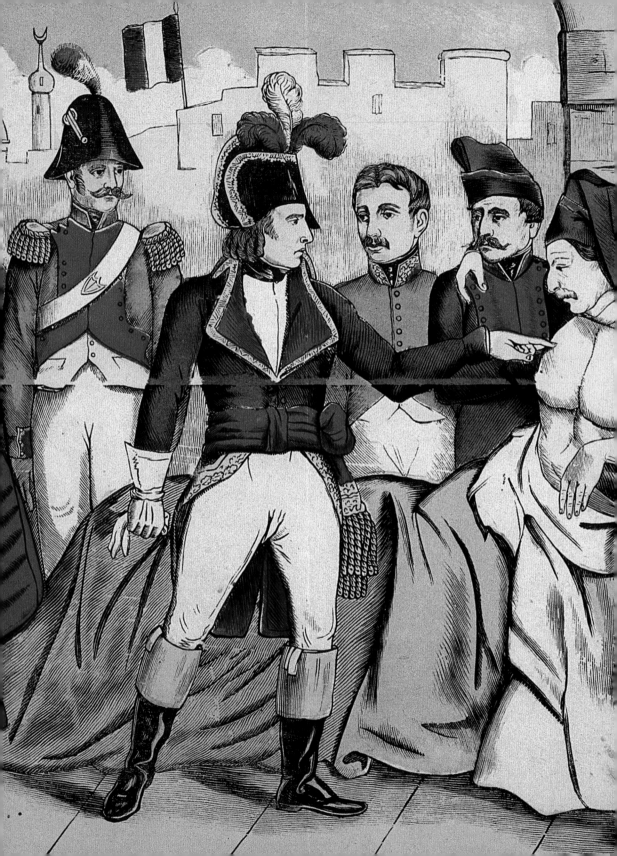

10
DOCTORS AT WAR: MILITARY MEDICINE FROM NAPOLEONIC TIMES

War and medicine make strange bedfellows, locked in an apparently antithetical embrace. But this marriage of opposites has been a mutually beneficial creative relationship: effective medicine reduces casualties, restores men to the battlefield and raises morale; war drives technical progress and provides doctors with large numbers of potential and actual patients for investigation and experimentation. The history of warfare marches in step with the Wellcome collections from the Middle Ages onwards, but perhaps no period is as colourfully illuminated as the period of almost continuous conflict between the French Revolution and the fall of Napoleon.

A mong the prodigious number of French historical artefacts and documents acquired by Sir Henry Wellcome and his chief continental agent, Captain Johnston-Saint (for which both were awarded the Légion d'Honneur), was a small collection of papers of René Desgenettes (1762–1837), physician in chief of the Egyptian expedition, 1798–1801.[1] Desgenettes published his own account of the expedition, *Histoire médicale de l'Armée d'Orient* (Paris, 1802), upon his return to France, largely based on his own letters, of which he seems to have kept copies. The letters now in the Wellcome collection are a selection of those sent to him, to which he also had access in writing his book. They provide a tangible sense of the expedition as it unfolded in a way that even contemporary printed works cannot hope to evoke.

Much effort was directed towards preventing the spread of plague: Desgenettes notes in his book the case of a storekeeper at Damietta, one of the first victims of the disease under the French occupation, which was referred to him because the local physicians could not agree on the cause of death. This report is among the Wellcome papers. Later in his book Desgenettes remarks that he had decided not to publish a most original letter from a Provençal cook, who offered Bonaparte a sure remedy for dysentery in the army – a mixture of hartshorn and the soft inside of a loaf of bread strained through a napkin and drunk warm – lest it detract from the seriousness of his work. This eccentrically spelt missive, forwarded by General Berthier to Desgenettes for his opinion, is also in the Wellcome collection.

Desgenettes left Egypt in the summer of 1801, following the capitulation of the French garrison to Lord Keith, presumably taking his papers with him. But another batch of papers relating to the Egyptian expedition had evidently fallen into British hands, since one of the documents is endorsed in a contemporary hand 'Sir Sidney Smith' (Sir William Sidney Smith, in command of HMS *Tigre*, which took part in the campaign).[2] These documents, which were purchased by Wellcome in London in 1919, include a copy of a decoded despatch from Bonaparte to the revolutionary government in Paris, of June 1799, referring to the high mortality among the expedition's doctors and the prevailing ignorance about local diseases.

Previous page:
Detail of a coloured wood engraving by Thiébault of Napoleon Bonaparte touching the bubo of a plague victim at Jaffa (Haifa) in 1799

Nelson's Navy

The fifteen bound volumes of administrative papers that document the command of the British Mediterranean fleet under Admiral Nelson between 1796 and 1805 do not relate exclusively, or even predominantly, to medicine, but they contain a lot of information about provisioning, sickness, naval hospitals and other matters that would have made them an attractive acquisition for Henry Wellcome.[3] They were purchased from a bookseller in 1928, having apparently been among the papers Nelson left in his house at Merton in September 1805 (there is nothing of later date than August 1805), when he left for the last time to rejoin the fleet prior to Trafalgar.

The overall impression conveyed by the papers is of remarkable administrative efficiency, not least in maintaining the health of seamen by ensuring adequate supplies of necessary foodstuffs, a challenge made all the more difficult by the closure of Spanish sources of provisions with that country's declaration of war on Britain in December 1804. The interruption of Spanish supplies coincided tellingly with a rise of scurvy in the fleet, which was only brought under control when alternative sources of fresh food were secured: John Snipe, the physician of the fleet, personally contracted with an English merchant at Messina to supply 10,000 gallons of freshly pressed Sicilian lemon juice.

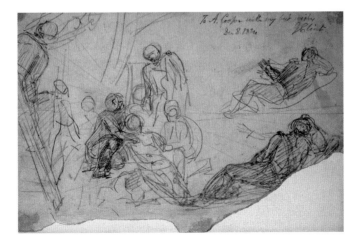

The death of Lord Nelson at the battle of Trafalgar, sketched by A. W. Devis on board HMS *Victory*, 1805

Napoleon's surgeon

Unquestionably the most glamorous Napoleonic figure represented in the Wellcome collections is Dominique Larrey (1766–1842), Napoleon's surgeon-in-chief. The collection contains his Leipzig campaign journal and a series of letters written to his wife and daughter between 1797 and 1814 that provide a commentary on Bonaparte's bloody campaigns.[4] Much of the correspondence was formerly in the renowned Napoleonic collection of Ludovic Lindsay, 26th Earl of Crawford, which was dispersed in the 1920s. Larrey published his own memoirs of the Napoleonic wars, *Mémoires de Chirurgie Militaires, et Campagnes* (Paris, 1812–17), but his letters connect us with an intimate lived experience that is all but edited out of the published work.

Despite his reputation and skill the letters make clear how dependent Larrey always was on the patronage and whim of Bonaparte: an Imperial decree abolishing travelling expenses for the officers of the Guard in autumn 1806 left Larrey high and dry in Prussia, borrowing money to be able to continue to accompany his Emperor, a decision on which he of course had no choice. A nice variation on the *Grande Armée*'s habit of living off the land is provided by several of Larrey's letters which are written on the Queen of Prussia's notepaper.

To perform a task as difficult as that which is imposed on a military surgeon, I am convinced one must often sacrifice oneself, perhaps entirely, to others, must scorn fortune, and must maintain an absolute integrity.

Dominique Larrey in his 1813 campaign journal
(translation courtesy of Robert Richardson)

The eternal struggle of the army doctor with the military authorities for the necessary means to do his job is a constant complaint, but it is lowly quartermasters and staff officers who bear the brunt of Larrey's scorn, rather than the real author of the French soldier's misfortunes: Napoleon himself remains a figure of veneration, whimsical and unpredictable, but ultimately unknowable and probably infallible. One of Larrey's letters to his wife describes the last days of Marshal Lannes, fatally wounded in 1809 at the battle of Wagram, whom Larrey attended to the end. Other letters are written from Russia, and give a first-hand account of the battle of Borodino and the burning of Moscow in 1812.

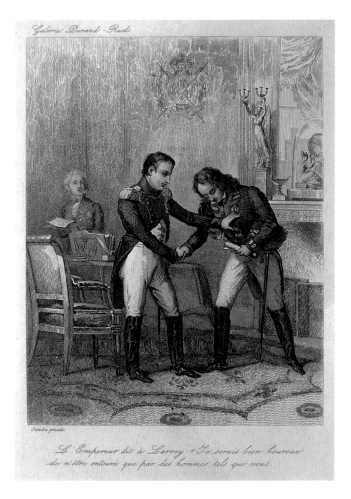

An engraving of Napoleon's surgeon-in-chief, Dominique Larrey, receiving the Emperor's congratulations in 1813

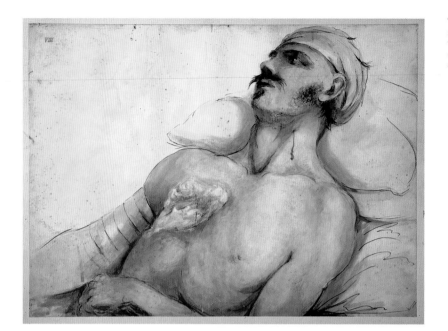

Two watercolours from
sketches of soldiers
wounded at the battle
of Waterloo, 1815, by the
surgeon Sir Charles Bell

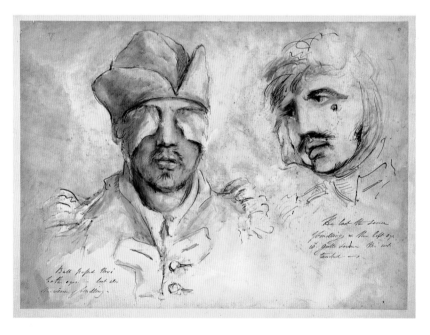

The Battle of Waterloo

None of Larrey's letters describes Waterloo, though he served there and famously was noticed by Wellington. Other documents in the Wellcome Library, however, provide unique windows on to the carnage of the battle. Probably the best-known are the watercolours of wounded soldiers by Sir Charles Bell (1774–1842) in the Royal Army Corps Muniment collection, which has been held in the Wellcome Library since 1991.[5] Bell had hurried from London to Brussels in June 1815 to assist in treating the wounded. As he did so he filled a sketchbook with interesting cases which he subsequently worked up as watercolour paintings for teaching purposes (sadly the original sketches, which were formerly kept on the open shelves of the Royal Army Medical School Library, were stolen in about 1930 and have never been recovered).

We have had lots of legs and arms to lop off.

From a letter from Isaac James, army surgeon treating the wounded of Waterloo, to his brother, Brussels, 29 June 1815

Also in the RAMC Muniments is a small collection of letters written to Bell by army surgeons in Brussels, after he had returned to London.[6] They describe the ongoing treatment of several cases of interest to Bell in terms that clearly illustrate what an unparalleled opportunity a major battle provided for surgical observation, research and experiment. The surgeons look forward to publication of some of the cases in the medical literature, and the letters strongly imply that the cross-Channel rush of British medical men to Brussels on hearing news of the battle of Waterloo was not entirely driven by altruism.

WAR AND MEDICINE
RELATED COLLECTIONS

The RAMC Muniment collection is the largest and most important collection in the Wellcome Library for the history of military medicine. This collection, which belongs to the Trustees of the Army Medical Services Museum, comprises correspondence, reports, diaries, photographs and a wealth of other documentation relating to the medical history of the British army, from the eighteenth century to the Falklands War. The old-fashioned term 'muniment' has been retained to describe this collection as it usefully serves to distinguish it from the official records of the RAMC held in the National Archives.

It is far from being a predictable archival entity that follows the history of the RAMC in a coherent way. It contains elements you might expect to find in the public records, such as the records of the Pathological Board in the Crimea,[7] or the correspondence and reports of William Fergusson (1773–1846), Inspector of Army Hospitals in Portugal during the Peninsular War.[8] But it is also a kaleidoscopic assemblage of documentation illuminating all aspects of British military medicine over three centuries. The earliest document is a draft letter of appointment of Charles II's surgeon-general, 1657.[9] The most up-to-date acquisitions are perhaps four photographs of a visit in June 1987 by the Dunkirk Veterans Association to war graves in France.[10]

Civilians in uniform

The major wars involving the British army during the twentieth century were the only wars in British military history fought mainly by civilians in uniform rather than by professional soldiers. The RAMC (which was not formed until 1898) expanded hugely during both World Wars to reflect the size of the citizen armies it served and to accommodate large numbers of civilian doctors and orderlies. And since civilians in uniform are more likely than professional soldiers to regard their wartime experiences as exceptional, they are also perhaps keener to record and preserve them.

There is consequently much more documentation in the Muniment collection for these periods than for any other. The papers of Hugh Glyn-Hughes (1892–1973), for instance, are of outstanding interest and importance. Covering his service between 1915 and 1945, they comprise a range of official and private documentation and include photographs of the retreat to Dunkirk and the liberation of Belsen.[11] Sir John Smith Knox Boyd (1891–1981), who was a regular rather than a volunteer, had an exceptionally significant military medical career and his papers provide important documentation on army blood transfusion, enteric fevers, tetanus immunisation and other matters in the Second World War.[12]

These poor unfortunates were reduced to frightened, inarticulate children ... a high proportion still exhibited signs of terror when approached and it was painful to watch one of the first batches of patients who had been selected for X-rays of chest. They struggled, cried and screamed as if they were being taken away for some form of torture.

Report by Major R. J. Phillips, Adviser in Psychiatry, Second Army, Belsen concentration camp, 1945, from the papers of Brigadier Hugh Glyn-Hughes

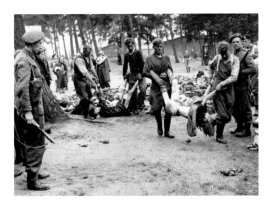

A photograph of concentration camp victims at the liberation of Belsen in April 1945, from the papers of Brigadier Hugh Glyn-Hughes

THE MEMORY OF A MILITARY HOSPITAL

by Philip Hoare

In the spring of 2000, while working on what was to become my book, *Spike Island*, I had become frustrated by the paucity of primary source material to document the vast Victorian hospital at Netley which was my subject. Set on the banks of Southampton Water, and built during the Crimean War, Netley was an imperial edifice one quarter of a mile long. It served the Empire for a hundred years, but since its demolition in 1966, it appeared to have vanished from the historical record. There were barely eleven items from Netley in the Public Record Office, for instance.

I was delighted, then, to discover that the Wellcome had a substantial collection of papers belonging to Sir Thomas Longmore, Netley's first Professor of Military Surgery. Longmore was one of a procession of figures from the hospital who retained an individuality which its vastness indulged and even encouraged – as if its hundreds of rooms gave free rein to their eccentricities, their triumphs and their mistakes.

Longmore, the son of a Royal Navy surgeon, had served in the Crimean War; his experiences there made him a leading authority: his 1861 publication, *Gunshot Wounds*, was required reading for surgeons in the American Civil War. Three years later Longmore became the British Representative at the first Geneva Convention. By then, he was already established as Professor of Military Surgery at Netley.

Longmore's papers detail many cases, but none more remarkable than that of Major Robert Hackett. Fighting in the Zulu Wars in South Africa, Hackett had received a bullet straight through his head. The missile entered one temple, exited on the other. Amazingly, he survived – although it was left to Longmore, who cared for Hackett back at Netley – to inform the officer that his blindness was permanent.

'Unfortunately this does not appear to have been made clear to the patient, so that on his arrival at Netley he still had a hope that he might recover the sight of one eye. It has been explained to Major Hackett how baseless this hope is & he has received the information, which it has been painful to communicate to him, with composure.' Humane as they were, Longmore's observations seemed almost surreal. 'The sense of smell is much impaired. Major Hackett can smell a flower for example, but he cannot distinguish between the odour of a rose & a carnation.' Elsewhere, his papers produced illustrations of wounded soldiers stitched up like Frankenstein's monsters.

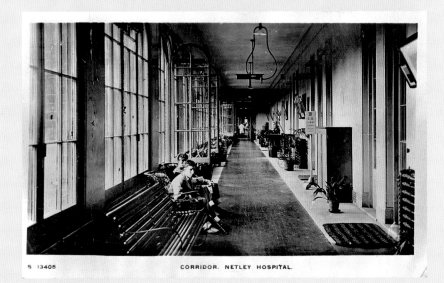

S 13405   CORRIDOR. NETLEY HOSPITAL.

The long corridor at Netley in 1910

Netley went on to nurture other mavericks: Almroth Wright, who trialled his anti-typhoid vaccine on himself and his own young officers; and later, R. D. Laing, who served in Netley's military asylum – the first of its kind, where Wilfred Owen, among thousands of others, was treated for shell shock. There Laing would evolve the theories which led to his book, *The Divided Self*. For these stories, and many others, I must be thankful to Wellcome and its archivists who daily delivered boxes to my desk in that hushed room on the Euston Road, each one, it seemed, containing something more extraordinary than the last.

❖

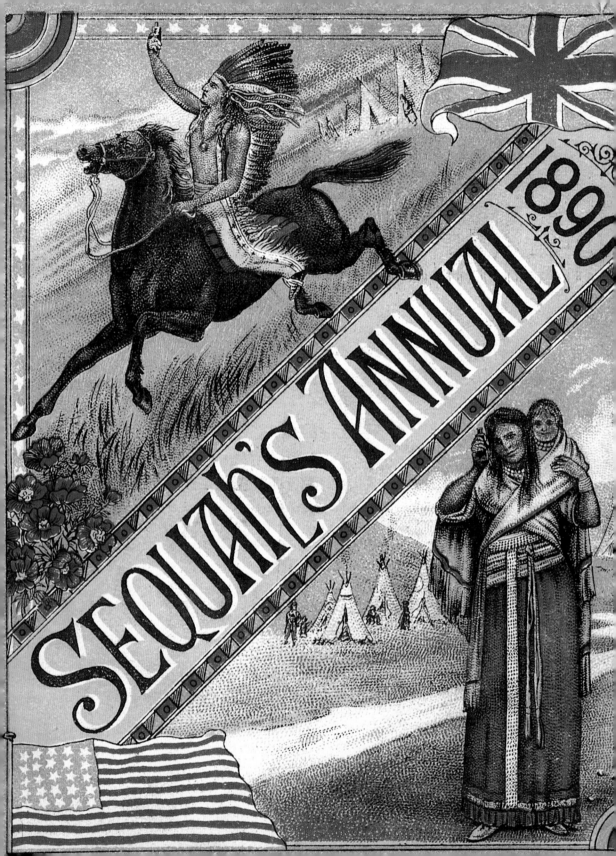

SEQUAH'S ANNUAL

1890

II
A QUICK FIX: PROPRIETARY MEDICINES AND THEIR PURVEYORS

Complementary therapies and alternative medicine currently enjoy an unprecedented respectability. A growing recognition of the potential benefits of non-conventional therapies among members of the orthodox medical profession has been accompanied by increasing interest in personal wellbeing, enhanced access to healthcare information and widespread availability of products. But it was not ever thus. The historical relationship between the orthodox and the unqualified practitioner is fraught with disagreement, condemnation and litigation. A hundred years ago the *British Medical Journal* printed a series of articles in which the hidden contents of 'miraculous' cures such as Box's Golden Fire ('The Quint-essence of Life!') and Wallace's Specific Remedies (deemed to be a 'a pretty specimen of "absolute" nonsense') were divulged – much to the chagrin of the manufacturers. But the purveyors of proprietary remedies were not prepared to give up their lucrative business without a fight.

Eye-catching advertisements, impressive showmanship and a reputation for results were three of the weapons in the armoury of proprietary drug merchants. They targeted the ills that orthodox practitioners failed to overcome and claimed astonishing cures. Some advertising campaigns were accompanied by a subtle denigration of the medical profession, while others proudly proclaimed the use that doctors made of their products. Brand identity was an essential element of the marketing strategy and was fiercely protected, with consumers being urged to check the authenticity of the products they purchased. The Sequah archive in the Archives and Manuscripts collections at the Wellcome Library brings together letters, advertisements and account books of a relatively successful but short-lived proprietary drug company towards the end of the nineteenth century.[1]

The modern physician, although he may be a man of learning and culture; although he may have so complete a knowledge of anatomy as to be able to describe the most insignificant bone or muscle in the body; although he may have completely mastered the signs or symptoms of every complaint incident to the human frame; although he may have practised for long years in the hospital wards or at the private bedside, is still almost entirely ignorant on the very point he is generally supposed and expected to be most proficient: he does not know how to cure disease.

A letter from W. H. Hartley, aka Sequah, in the *Edinburgh Evening Dispatch*, 12 December 1888

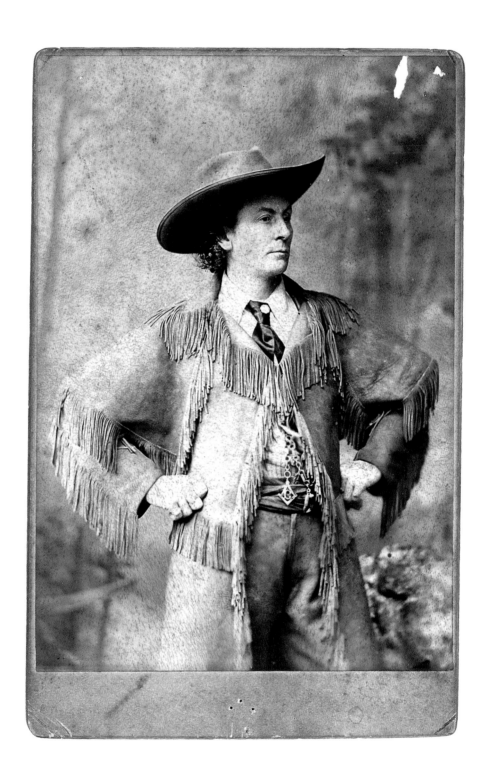

Who and what was Sequah?

Sequah's cures were marketed through a roadshow which was conducted with all the razzmatazz of the American medicine shows which inspired it. The arrival of one of about twenty-five 'Sequahs' (at the peak of its operation) was announced by a raucous procession with a brass band and bass drummer drawn through the streets on a colossal gold chariot. Posters and handbills announcing that the great Sequah had arrived were distributed to the gathering crowd. Curious onlookers attracted by the band were invited to one of two daily performances that the famed medicine man would be giving. At the designated time a horse-drawn wagon would drive up to the chosen location, generally a circus ground, open field or marketplace. Sequah had arrived. Tall, sporting a large, broad-brimmed Stetson hat and attired Red Indian-style in a buckskin coat and leggings, he spoke with a pronounced American accent as he enthralled the crowd with accounts of his travels in the Wild West and his desire to ease the suffering of humanity through his Indian botanic remedies.

The band struck up a lively tune while Sequah displayed his expertise in drawing teeth 'free, gratis and for nothing' (as the promotional booklet *Who and what is Sequah?* proclaimed) for a queue of willing volunteers. American dentists were then widely regarded as being at the top of their profession and Sequah was no slouch, performing at great speed with an electric lamp attached to his forehead and a fine array of dentistry instruments. This was followed by a demonstration of the near-miraculous healing powers of his two main products. A swig of 'Prairie Flower' followed by a vigorous massage of 'Indian Oil', conducted by Sequah with the help of a number of cowboy and American Indian assistants, would restore mobility to a sufferer from incurable rheumatism. The outcome was so remarkable, according to accounts, that patients had been known to celebrate their recovery by breaking into a dance. The two products would then go on sale for a while, but not for too long, since many punters had to be sent away empty-handed in order to ensure their return for the next show. Sequah would remain in town until the novelty wore off and the income fell away; then the roadshow would move on in search of pastures new.

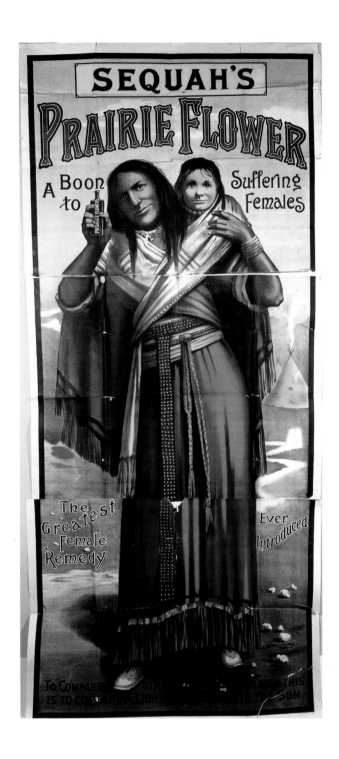

A Sequah advertisement exploiting the 'Red Indian' mystique, c. 1890

Advertisements in the Sequah archive refer to the 'peerless' capabilities of the two main remedies which professed to cure not only rheumatism and 'impure blood' but also asthma, bronchitis, boils, blotches, influenza, catarrh, dyspepsia, glandular swellings, hives, itch, and all diseases arising from an inactive liver. Posters emphasised the generosity of Sequah, who gave away remedies free of charge to the deserving poor, while booklets carried glowing references, notably from members of the clergy. The marketing highlight, however, was the weekly *Sequah Chronicle*, which combined an all-out advertising campaign with flattering reports of the various Sequahs' visits to towns across the country.

The subject under treatment became very fidgety and uneasy; he groaned, he wriggled and struggled to regain his liberty, but the cowboys, thinking that these were merely indications of a shrinking will under the painful ordeal, and that the man would recover his steadfastness of purpose, hurried on with the cure so that it should be short as well as sharp ... the subject, however, gradually became more uneasy; he struggled frantically; he bellowed for relief; then he prayed for deliverance from his supposed torturers with such intensity and such evident dread that Sequah gave the order to desist ...

From a report in the *Liverpool Echo*, 11 August 1890

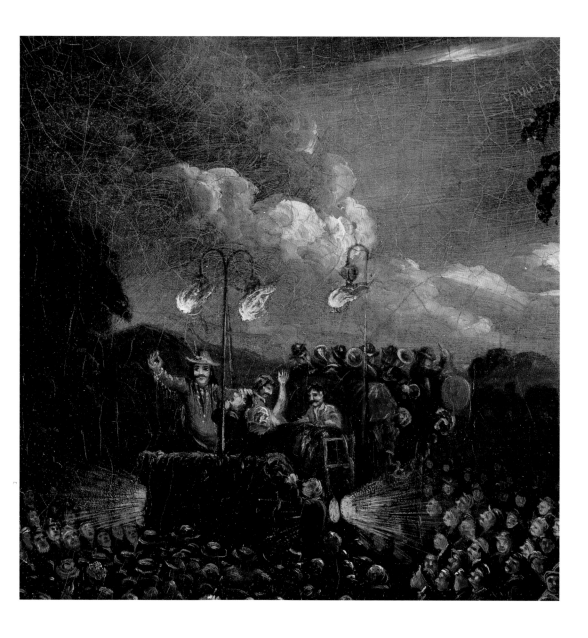

Detail from an oil
painting, c. 1890, of the
Sequah roadshow on
Clapham Common

'James Kasper'

The diaries, accounts and correspondence of Peter Alexander Gordon provide another view of the operation of Sequah Ltd. Originally operating as a clairvoyant, Gordon performed under the stage name of James Kasper and was employed by the company between 1890 and 1892. His correspondence with William Hartley, the original Sequah and founder of Sequah Ltd., illuminates the company's endeavours to expand its international horizons following the UK Customs and Inland Revenue Act 1890, which banned the sale of proprietary medicines from mobile chariots (or a stage) and effectively ended its operations in Britain.

Remember that you never do your work right on one of these wagons until your shirt is wet, and when you have perspired sufficiently to wet your shirt so that you can take it off and ring it out, then you have done your duty. As you feel, so do the people feel, and if you do not warm yourself up you will never warm the people up. You must work with a will and heart, and make them understand that you are interested in what you are doing and that you believe in the merits of the goods you are selling with your whole heart, body, soul and mind.

A letter from W. H. Hartley to James Kasper, 22 September 1890

A combination of letters, cargo invoices and account books charts Kasper's journey through the Caribbean, Canada and Spain, providing a vivid description of the competition he faced from vendors of rival brands. Even before he had arrived in Georgetown, Guyana, one competitor was attempting to undermine his operation by sending a letter to the local authorities accusing him of being an impostor. A different kind of challenge came with the discovery that his assistant, who perhaps subscribed to the 'no honour among thieves' code, had been secretly supplying his rivals with unbranded supplies of Sequah's remedies which they then passed off as their own products.

Kasper eventually fell out with Hartley and on his return to England he deposited his box of papers in the Birkbeck Bank in London. This bank was liquidated in 1911, after which the papers were removed to the vaults of the Bank of England. There they remained undisturbed until 1982 when – once they had been opened and their intrinsic historical interest established – they were presented to the Wellcome Library.

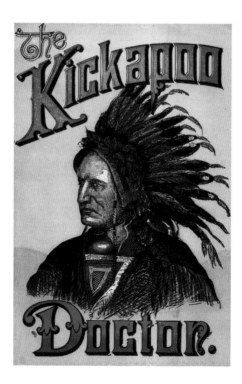

Advertisement for the Kickapoo Doctor, a rival company to Sequah, c. 1890

ALTERNATIVE MEDICINE
RELATED COLLECTIONS

The Sequah archive provides a perfect illustration of the type of
alternative medicine that orthodox practitioners hoped to eradicate.
It does not, however, typify alternative medicine or complementary
therapies as they are understood today, when research is undertaken
not so much to expose them as to assess their potential benefits. While
mainstream medicine may not exactly embrace its less orthodox
neighbours, the path is set for further interaction and cooperation.
Some forms of alternative medicine have shed the 'unqualified' label
and gained respectability by introducing professional regulating
bodies, such as the British Osteopathic Association, whose archives
are also held in the library.[2]

   The British Medical Association's archive contains a selection of
letters, minutes from meetings of the ethical committee and excerpts
from newspapers on proprietary medicine.[3] Two booklets, *Secret
Remedies: what they cost and what they contain* (1909) and *More Secret
Remedies: what they cost and what they contain* (1912), comprise the
series of articles originally published in the *British Medical Journal*
and cited in the introduction to this chapter. The library's Ephemera
collections include four boxes of Herbal Medicine Ephemera, as well
as over a hundred boxes containing drug advertisements of both
orthodox and alternative proprietary remedies.[4] Then there is the
Wellcome Library's unrivalled Asian collection of books, manuscripts
and artefacts expounding eastern systems of health like ayurveda
and techniques such as acupuncture.

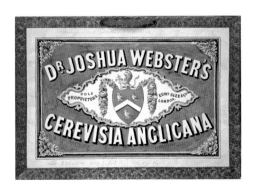

The Slee familiy's
advertisement for
Dr Webster's Diet Drink,
formulated in 1742

Portrait of Dr Joshua
Webster in 1801, aged 92

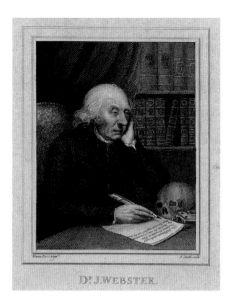

Dr J.WEBSTER.

Dr Webster's Diet Drink

In 1994 the Wellcome purchased the surviving papers of a
Southwark wine and spirit merchant with the splendidly Dickensian
name of Samuel Slee.[5] He and his descendants were the proprietors
of a Georgian universal remedy known as Dr Webster's Diet Drink.
This medicine reportedly had been formulated in 1742 by Joshua
Webster (1709?–1801), who claimed to have cured Benjamin
Franklin of a scorbutic complaint with his diet drink and ascribed his
own longevity to occasional doses of the medicine. The collection is
mainly a record of the exploitation of the recipe and Webster's
reputation by the Slee family throughout the nineteenth century.

The recipe, of course, was a closely guarded secret, and no clue
as to the particular ingredients was given on the 'octagon square
shaped red and green bottles' in which the drink was sold, though
females were warned to avoid it 'at certain times'. It was promoted
as a non-specific remedy of vegetable extraction, and the fact that it
contained mercury did not prevent the proprietors from warning
customers against 'mercurial quacks'. In the cut-throat market for
health, as much as in war, truth was the first casualty.

GOIGS DE SANT CLEMENT PA-
PA, Y MARTIR, PA- TRÒ DE LA ESPUNYO
la Bisbat de Solsona.

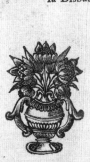

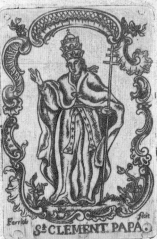

Ferriols fecit
St CLEMENT PAPA.

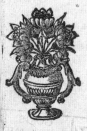

Puix vostre nom nos combida
à pregarvos humilment:
siau clement ab qui u's crida,
Papa, y Martir Sant Clement.

En Roma noble Ciutat
del rich Faustino nasquereu;
pero mes noble la fereu
ab vostra gran santedat:
de Sant Pere sou estàt
deixeble lo mes eminent. Siau, &c.

Ja de deixeble passareu
à ser Mestre universal,
puix la Cathedra Papal,
en ella sentàt honràreu:
dels Sants Martirs il·lustràreu
las hazanyas sabiament: &c.

Vostra singular doctrina,
que honra à la Iglesia donà,
à innumerables portà
Gentils à la Fè Divina:
vostra ploma peregrina
al Cel donà lluiment: &c.

La deserta soledàt,
hont Trajano vos desterra,
ab vos en poblada terra
en un instant se ha mudàt:
perque anàu acompanyat
de un sens numero de gent: &c.

Patint la gent sed estranya,
en una font aigua beù,
que un anyell formà ab lo pèu
en lo coll de una montanya:
esta fou insigne hazanya
de vostra oració fervent: &c.

Aquella aigua prodigiosa
à molts Infiels convertì,
y de Sant vos adquirì
nom, respecte, y fama honrosa:
mes vostre zel no reposa
en donar à la Fè aument: &c.

La tirania irritada
de tants miracles, ordena,
que en vostre coll ab cadena
sia una anchora lligada:
vostra vida aixi llançada
fou al salobre Element: &c.

Los Christians ab llibertat
dintre del mar sens entraren,
perque sas onas deixàren
pas franch à la pietàt:
tal miracle ha publicàt
vostre merit excel·lent: &c.

Un Temple miraculòs,
que Angels en marbre labràren,

dintre de la mar trobàren
y en una arca vostre cos:
la esperança mes patent: &c.

Publicas aclamacions
aquella terra u's donà
y la lley infiel deixà
de falsas adoracions:
de singulars conversions
viu, y mort sou instrument: &c.

Del Poble de la Espunyola
sou nùvol acreditat,
puix en temps de sequedat
per vos la pluja lo consola:
à vostra clemencia vòla
en tot perill imminent: &c.

També sòu font de salut,
que curàu las malaltias,
sempre que ab pregarias pias
à vos han recorregùt:
los Forasters, que han vingut,
han curat en continent: &c.

TORNADA.
Puix la Espunyola u's adora
per son Patró, y Advocat:
Sant Clement Martir Sagrat,
amparau·lo en tota hora.

℣. Justus ut palma florebit. ℟. Sicut Cedrus Libani multiplicabitur.

OREMUS

Deus, qui nos annua beati Clementis martyris tui, atque Pontificis solemnitate lætificas: Concede propitius; ut cujus natalitia colimus, virtutem quoque passionis imitemur. Per Christum, &c.

Lo Ill.m y Rm. Sr. D. Fr. Joseph de Mezquia Bisbe de Solsona conced 40. dias de Indulgencia per cada Cobla que llegiràn, ohiràn llegir, ò cantar de estos Goigs, y tanbe 40. per cada Pare nostre, Ave Maria, y Gloria Patri, &c. se diràn à Sant Clement.

12
GOIGS AND THANKAS: THE BENIGN AND MALIGN IN CATALONIA AND TIBET

One of the purposes of Henry Wellcome's collections, like most historical collections, is to assist understanding of our own situation by placing it against the backdrop of the wider world, and particularly against the larger historical context provided by ancient and alien cultures. The search for health through medical knowledge – to take one important subject in the collections – appears to be one of the means by which human beings attempt to preserve themselves from danger and destruction. Such strivings take many forms, and the explorer in the Wellcome Library will encounter some of the more exotic guises in which they appear in different periods and places. Two examples of such expressions in the library's iconographic collections are the Catalonian prints called *goigs*, which provide a means of communication between human beings and benevolent sacred beings of Christian faith; and, in Tibetan Buddhism, portable paintings – *thankas* in Tibetan – some of which also invoke benevolent deities, while others serve to appease horrific malign forces.

*G*oigs is a Catalan word, equivalent to *gozos* in Castilian and *gaudia* in Latin: they all mean rejoicings, things to rejoice about, or causes of rejoicing. However, the word has a special meaning as applied to small sheets of paper about 30 x 20 cm, printed usually on one side with the following elements:

– At the top a print (usually a woodcut, lithograph or halftone, less commonly an intaglio print) of a sacred figure: Christ, the Virgin, a saint, or one of the Christian mysteries;
– a heading, in Catalan, identifying the figure, for example as a reproduction of a sacred painting or sculpture in a particular parish church in Catalonia;
– a hymn to be sung in procession or in congregation, in Catalan;
– a prayer to be intoned by a priest, in Latin.

Common additions to the printed matter include an indulgence and an imprint. The indulgence grants a specific number of days' remission of punishment for reciting prayers in the presence of the sacred effigy, while the imprint identifies the printer and the address from which the sheet could be bought. Occasionally there is a date of publication. Sometimes a musical score accompanies the words of the hymn. Often there are decorative borders and type ornaments, occasionally with hand-colouring.

Goigs are an essentially, and almost uniquely, Catalan genre, and their historical interest has long been recognised. Indeed it is only the diligence of *goig*-collectors of the past that enables us to say anything about *goigs* today. The *Asociación 'Amics dels Goigs'* was founded in 1854 and still publishes a quarterly *Butlletí*. Major collectors include the Barcelona antiquarian Don Salvador Babra; *el princeps dels goigistes* Dr Salvador Roca i Ballber, who owned 20,000 *goigs*; and, more recently, Josep Maria Gavín (b. 1930), founder of the Arxiu Gavín at Valldoreix, in the town of Sant Cugat del Vallés.

None was more enthusiastic than Father Lambert Botey, who not only collected *goigs* but was also responsible for commissioning some in his capacity as prior of the mediaeval Hospital de la Santa Creu in Barcelona. (Coincidentally, the hospital building is now the home of the Biblioteca de Catalunya, which also has a collection of *goigs*.) Botey's collection of *goigs* was bought by Henry Wellcome from the collector in 1928 as a result of one of Wellcome's collecting expeditions

Previous page:
Goig of St Clement (Pope Clement I) as patron saint of L'Espunyola, Catalonia. Mixed method incorporating an engraving by Ferriols and an indulgence by Fr Joseph de Mezquía (Bishop of Solsona 1746–72)

Opposite:
Detail of The Last Judgment. Coloured woodcut with letterpress published in Barcelona in 1858 by the heirs of the widow Pla

in northern Spain and the Pyrenees. The ex-Botey collection is preserved intact in the Wellcome Library today: it arrived in London in two large parcels in June 1928, spent most of the following sixty years in a filing cabinet, and has recently been transferred to 31 solander boxes. It is believed to be the only collection of *goigs* in the UK, and possibly the only major collection outside Catalonia. Botey credibly estimated it at about 6,000 sheets. Some of his *goigs* bear the ownership-stamps of earlier collectors (for example, Josep Duran and F. Martí), but the extent to which he absorbed earlier collections has yet to be ascertained. Cataloguing of the Wellcome Library *goigs* at an item-by-item level has a long way to go before it reaches the level of the Biblioteca de Catalunya, which has descriptions of about a thousand *goigs* in its online catalogue.

Negotiating with cosmic forces

The subjects of the Wellcome *goigs* include both standard themes of Catholic devotion, such as the Ecce Homo and the Virgin of the Seven Sorrows, and many more unusual subjects, such as Christ crucified on the walnut tree; the unofficial but very useful saint Expeditus; the Last Judgment; and local appeals for intervention against drought and hailstorms. Against epidemics the most popular resort is to the

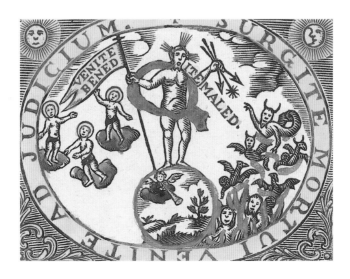

mediaeval plague saints Sebastian and Roch, less often to Christopher. Successful childbirth is commonly requested in *goigs* of the Virgin. The Passion is commemorated as the exemplar of bodily suffering inevitably entailed by God's assumption of human form in Jesus Christ. Such prints could be used in procession, in church, or privately: one account describes how an adulterous woman intent on suicide was saved from herself by looking on the printed image of Christ, while others report relief of pain when the sacred sheet was pressed against an injured part.

On the other side of the globe, in Tibet, there are also cultural means for humans to negotiate with cosmic forces, and one of these is the *thanka* or portable painting (as distinct from a wall-painting or rock-painting). *Thanka* is also transliterated in English as *tanka*, *tangka*, and *thangka*. Wellcome's Tibetan paintings were mostly acquired in the 1920s in the London rooms of four different auction houses: Foster's, Glendining's, Stevens's and Sotheby's. Before their appearance at auction some had belonged to Lawrence Austine Waddell (1854–1938), a Scottish medical man and member of the Younghusband Mission of 1903–04, in which British soldiers invaded Tibet in order to demonstrate to Russia that Britain was determined to protect India's northern frontiers. Waddell's particular interest was Tibetan Buddhism, and Buddhist documents acquired by him in Tibet are today in several libraries in India and Great Britain. After his return from Tibet he was appointed Professor of Tibetan at University College London, and wrote several, still useful, books on Tibetan Buddhism.

Like *goigs*, Tibetan *thankas* also include specific defining elements. They are painted in distemper (pigments dissolved in a medium of rabbit glue) on cloth. The painting usually contains a large central figure of the Sakyamuni Buddha, a *bodhisattva*, or one of the other sacred Buddhist beings, placed against a coloured background and surrounded by smaller related figures. The painted cloth is laid down on a mount of patterned woven fabric. Attached along the top and bottom edges of the mount are wooden rods: when unrolled the work is suspended from the top rod, and when it is not on display it is rolled around the bottom one. A yellow silk wrap protects the painting from damage when rolled up. Many of the Wellcome paintings follow this standard pattern, and it is easy to appreciate that the tranquil, brightly painted deities provide a cheering or consoling presence to the

Bhaisajyaguru (above) and Padmasambhava (below, centre, with his consorts Mandarava and Yeshe Tsogyal). Distemper painting on cloth, Tibet, pre-1900

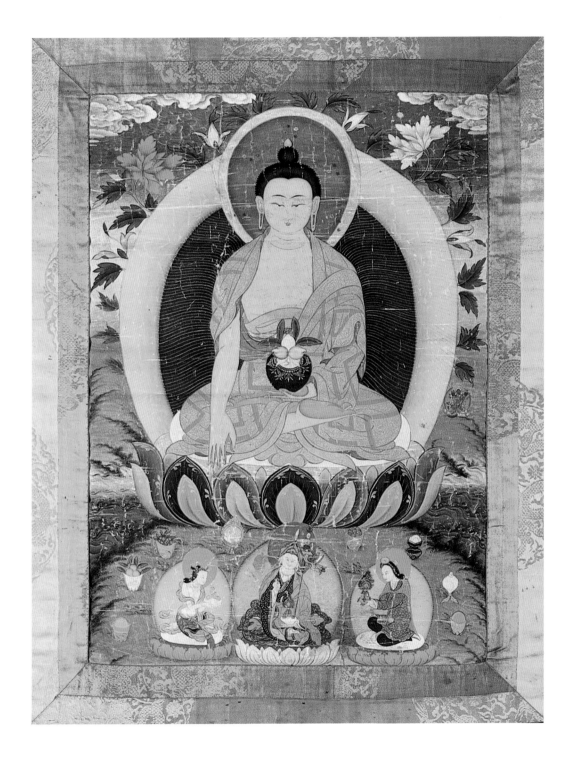

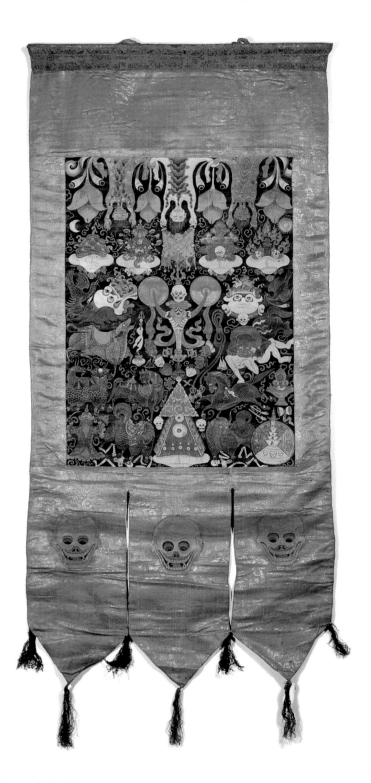

Attributes of
Yama Dharmarāja
(Yama Dam-can
Chos-kyi rGyal-po).
Distemper painting on
cloth, Tibet, pre-1900

worshipper distressed by hunger, pain, bereavement, or invasion by foreign powers. When many are displayed together, lit by shafts of sunlight falling through a temple doorway, the array of multicoloured figures creates an overwhelming vision of otherworldly splendour.

Protective messages

On the other hand, there are also paintings which anticipate the worst and try to prevent it. Unlike the serene and sunny world of the typical Tibetan painting, these grim works display human hides, necklaces of skulls, lions chewing human entrails, and mutilated body parts, all depicted against a sombre background in an effort to propitiate irate and savage demons. There are works from two such series in the Wellcome Library: one series comes, presumably via Waddell, from Palkhor Choedeh (dPal-'khor Chos-sde) Temple at Gyantse, while the iconography of the other series suggests an origin in Drepung or Lhasa. One of these is addressed to Yama, the Buddhist god of death, who sends disease and old age to human beings and acts as judge in the underworld. In these works the god himself is not shown for fear of making matters worse: instead we foresee in the painting the tortures to which he will consign us if we have sinned. The tone is set by the figures along the top edge, where skins of three flayed human beings alternate with bouquets of viscera, garnished with ripped-out eyes on stalk-like optic chiasmata.

Goigs and *thankas* have been studied from the point of view of local history and as works of art. Henry Wellcome's open-minded collecting policy draws them into a wider context, in which their function as protective messages comes to the fore. Conversely, those acquainted with the technology of biomedicine – especially surgery and pharmaceuticals – can be led, through Wellcome's collection, to the discovery that, for people of other cultures and periods, the culturally suggested route to tranquillity and wellbeing may be through a *goig*, a *thanka*, music or a book of spiritual healing. The Wellcome Library is one of the few institutions in which such a stimulating range of documents can be brought together from opposite sides of the Earth for scholars studying in the same room.

MAKING HONEY

by Sarah Bakewell

A book cataloguer's life is like that of a laser barcode-reader at a supermarket checkout. Many things pass the beam of your attention, but every so often something snags. No matter which way you look at it, it refuses to go through. If someone doesn't snatch the item away from you with a 'tut!' (which, I'm glad to say, rarely happens at the Wellcome), you can puzzle away happily until you make sense of it.

I catalogued books for the Wellcome Library for ten fascinating years. One of the first books to cross my desk was a 1930s compilation, *Chinese Materia Medica*. Among its remedies it included an account of certain Middle Eastern ascetics who used to starve themselves to death on a diet of honey alone. When they died, their bodies were sealed inside casks of more honey to macerate for a hundred years. The casks were then opened and the treacly substance inside dispensed as a panacea. The story is of dubious authenticity, but it appealed to me – perhaps because I like honey. I passed the cataloguing job to the Oriental department, but not the story, which stayed in my mind and started me researching the real history of *mumia*, or mummy medicine.

That was the first of many books to distract me from my job. Later, cataloguing an assortment of eighteenth-century pamphlets on various subjects, I came upon an entertaining diatribe called *Mrs Stewart's Case*. The author was furious with a Lord Rawdon, who had supported her for a while believing her to be a relative, but had stopped payments after hearing rumours about her true identity. No other information was given, not even her full name, which I needed for the record. I checked her out and found that 'Mrs Stewart' was one of a dozen pseudonyms belonging to the con artist Margaret Caroline Rudd. She had recently emerged scot-free from a forgery case which had seen her accomplices hanged – identical twin brothers, who died hand in hand on the gallows. Yet everyone (except herself) agreed that she was the mastermind behind the crime.

I dug for more, switching to working in my own time as the plot thickened, and ended up with so much material that it became a book, *The Smart*, a sort of non-fiction legal thriller. Of all the twists and surprises I encountered along the way, perhaps the most unexpected was that she really was related to Lord Rawdon.

Only a library such as the Wellcome generates such moments of serendipity. The atmosphere of freedom, curiosity and scholarship is just right, as is the sheer wealth of the collection itself – for it is a collection that resists categorisation, while remaining devoted to medicine in the fullest sense of the word.

It is wonderful to see its riches emerging into the light. Still, if some treasures lurk in the depths for a century or more, no matter. They may fester a little, but one day they will make honey for someone.

❖

Margaret Caroline Rudd in Newgate prison, 1776

C.B.C.

CONSTRUCTIVE

BIRTH CONTROL
SOCIETY AND FREE CLINIC

Founded by
DR. MARIE STOPES.

The Free Clinic is under the patronage of a distinguished Committee, staffed with qualified Lady Doctors and Certified Midwives.

The C.B.C. Headquarters are the Pioneer Centre for advice, instruction, and help.

108, Whitfield Street, W.1.   **Telephone: Museum 9528**

READ THE
BIRTH CONTROL NEWS

SIXPENCE MONTHLY.

Ask for it at the Railway Bookstalls

13
WIVES, LOVERS AND MOTHERS: SEX AND BIRTH CONTROL IN THE UK

During the twentieth century, limiting family size came to seem increasingly essential for economic reasons within the family, in the interest of women's health, and in the light of a global population explosion placing pressure on finite resources. In addition, a good sex life has come to be seen as important to healthy functioning. These developments are reflected in the largest single collection in the Wellcome Library's Archives and Manuscripts, that of the Family Planning Association, and in several related collections. The interest of this important archive extends well beyond the provision of birth control clinics.

The National Birth Control Association (NBCA) was established in 1930 by several bodies already working to promote the provision of birth control in the UK (the name was changed to Family Planning Association in 1939).[1]

Marie Stopes (1880–1958) is probably the name that springs to mind in association with the rise of an articulate birth control movement in the 1920s. Stopes performed a valuable service in her propaganda work to publicise the cause. Although her famous manual of marital sexual instruction, *Married Love*, published in 1918, only mentioned birth control as a possibility, later the same year she published a short lucid guide to the current methods of contraception called *Wise Parenthood*. Though her initial interest was in enabling couples (and in particular wives) to enjoy sexually fulfilling marriages, much of the correspondence generated by *Married Love* (thousands of these letters are now held in the Wellcome Library) was specifically about birth control, since the shadow of unwanted conception affected many. It is clear from reports by numerous correspondents that even when doctors were not hostile towards contraception they knew very little about the subject.[2]

I have by the greatest exercise of self-denial kept our family down to three, without any artificial checks, but it has been a great trial.

From a letter to Marie Stopes, undated, c. 1920s

Stopes and her second husband Humphrey Roe, himself a strong advocate of birth control, therefore established both an organisation, the Society for Constructive Birth Control, to campaign and to promote public awareness of contraception, and a flagship clinic, the Mothers' Clinic, in North London, to provide contraceptive advice to poor women. This clinic moved to Whitfield Street (off Tottenham Court Road) and is still the headquarters of Marie Stopes International. A number of provincial clinics were also set up with greater or lesser degrees of success, and Stopes also had the idea of a travelling 'Caravan Clinic'. She also produced the pamphlet, *A Letter to Working*

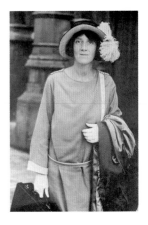

Previous page: `
A 1920s poster advertising the Society for Constructive Birth Control and Marie Stopes's free clinic

Above:
Marie Stopes leaving the law courts during her 1923 libel action

Opposite:
A nurse standing in front of Dr Marie Stopes's travelling caravan clinic, late 1920s

Mothers (1919 and much reissued), aimed at the poorer classes, and a textbook on *Contraception* (1923), since the medical profession were lagging in providing anything of this nature.

My wife and I have been married three years and we have not yet had a union, because we do not want children yet.

From a letter to Marie Stopes, undated, c. 1920s

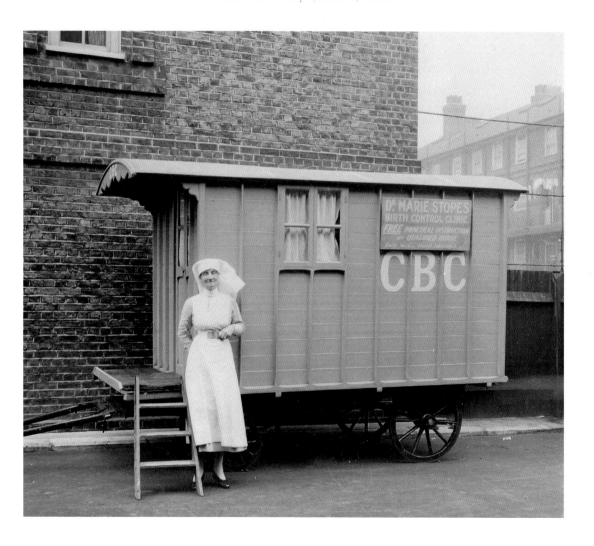

Stopes was also an adept user of the media. She was a newsworthy figure whose pronouncements often appeared in the press, as did interviews and articles. Her libel case against the Roman Catholic gynaecologist Halliday Sutherland, though it did not reach a satisfactory legal conclusion, was a successful piece of propaganda for her and for the birth control movement. But in spite of her high profile, which has tended to occlude fellow campaigners, she was far from being the only individual working for the promotion of birth control during the 1920s.

Shortly after she established the Mothers' Clinic, the Malthusian League founded the Walworth Women's Welfare Centre in South London: this eventually came under the management of the Society for the Provision of Birth Control Clinics, which set up a number of other clinics, including the North Kensington Clinic which undertook many pioneering initiatives. A number of other organisations were either setting up clinics, agitating for the Ministry of Health to permit birth control advice as part of rate-funded maternal welfare services, or beginning to conduct research on the efficacy of the methods available. However, when these existing organisations came together to unite their efforts as the NBCA in 1930, it was very difficult to persuade Stopes to join in, and she very shortly withdrew and maintained her independence.

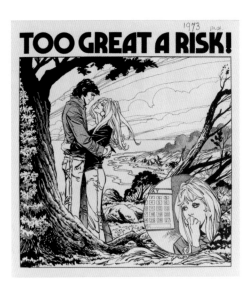

Family Planning Association leaflet, 1970s-style, by Gillian Crampton Smith

Eugenics and birth control

It has often been assumed by historians and others that the birth control movement was closely connected with contemporary notions about eugenics. But a reading of the literature produced both by individuals such as Stopes and by the movement as a whole suggests that issues of maternal welfare and personal happiness drove them much more strongly than fears about the 'unfit'. Even if people like Stopes made various public statements favourable to eugenics, this does not seem to have affected practice within clinics, which was about respecting the desires of the individual woman. Far from favouring birth control, the Eugenics Society of the UK feared that it was more likely to be used by the professional middle classes, whom they wanted to encourage to have larger families, rather than by the 'unfit'.[3] By the 1930s the Society, largely under the influence of Dr C. P. Blacker (1895–1975), whose papers are also in the Library,[4] may have come round to providing both rhetorical and financial support for birth control, but any influence they had on the agenda of the NBCA appears to have been minimal to say the least, while the new constitution that was drawn up at the time of the name-change to the Family Planning Association (FPA) made no reference whatsoever to eugenic arguments.

Most people probably think of the FPA as being predominantly about the provision of birth control clinics. Birth control was not incorporated into the National Health Service until 1974: thus the FPA was the main provider of clinics and also of specialised training for health professionals for a period of over forty years. It often experienced difficulty over advertising its clinics, as the subject was long considered verging on the obscene: London Transport famously refused to display a very bland poster as late as the 1950s.

Though there are copious records of clinics from all over the UK in the FPA archive, it was engaged in far more than merely running clinics. The NBCA had begun as a campaigning body trying to persuade the government to permit (though not require) local Medical Officers of Health to provide birth control advice in local authority maternity clinics to women who needed it. The FPA continued this lobbying and campaigning role, pressing successive governments to extend the grounds on which birth control could be given and to provide resources; it also put pressure on local authorities either to provide advice in their maternal welfare clinics, or to collaborate in establishing a birth control clinic.

I was very much afraid of my wife dying at one time and she has not got over it yet, so we dare not run any risk of having another … Finally I came out here [Nigeria] in the hope that both of us might get over our desires and be able to live together without being worried that way. That does not seem to have happened at all to either of us and while I want my wife to come out to me for a time very much, and she wants to come equally I dare not have her, nor dare I go home as things are.

From a letter to Marie Stopes, undated, c. 1920s

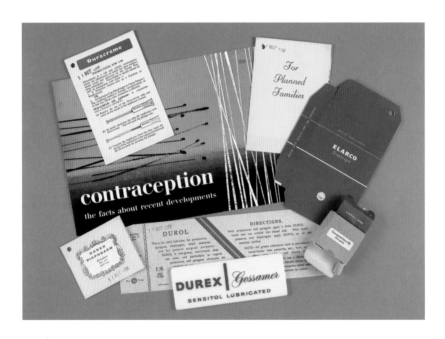

'Anything for the weekend, sir?' A selection of London Rubber Company products and material from the 1950s/1960s

Rubber johnnies and the Pill

The work of the Birth Control Investigation Committee, founded in 1927, in testing and evaluating commercially available contraceptives of the time, in order to ascertain which ones were safe and effective, was enthusiastically taken up by the NBCA. This involved building up good relationships with the manufacturers, who soon caught on that it was a valuable selling point to be on the Approved List. Some manufacturers, such as W. J. Rendell, with their Wife's Friend Pessaries, even claimed FPA approval for products that were not on the list. As a result the FPA archive contains an enormous amount of material relating to the manufacture of contraceptives – including the problems of rubber supply during the Second World War. There is also a huge quantity of extremely rare packaging, advertising and promotional material: one of the files for the London Rubber Company even incorporates examples of the discreet celluloid plaques for Durex products that were placed in the windows of chemists' or barbers' shops ('Anything for the weekend, sir?'). When the Pill was being developed in the late 1950s and early 1960s, clinical trials were coordinated by the FPA with the assistance of volunteer women recruited via the network of clinics.

Dr Voge criticized severely the condition of the condom market. Tests made from those purchased in the open market showed that only 55% were usable. The most usual practice was to test the article by the face-testing method which was very unreliable. The only safe method was the automatic one.

From the minutes of the NBCA Medical Sub-Committee, 1934

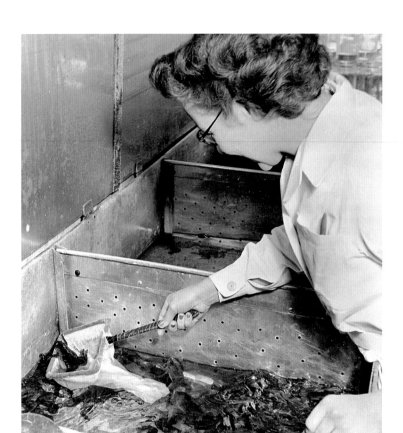

A laboratory worker
catching a xenopus toad,
used by the FPA for
pregnancy testing, c. 1950s

The FPA was not just about preventing babies; it also did
a good deal of work on the problems of low fertility, giving aid to
those who found it difficult to conceive. This meant involvement
in diagnosis as well as treatment. From the early 1940s one of
the services offered was artificial insemination. At a time when
pregnancy testing was not available over the counter, the FPA also
offered pregnancy testing, using xenopus toads. If a female toad
is injected with the urine of a pregnant woman, she lays eggs. This
was not only humane; it was an ecologically sound self-renewing
method, unlike the better known 'rabbit test', which involved killing
the rabbit. It also undertook what might be called more general
'well-woman' activities, such as providing cervical cytology tests.

Counselling and sex education

The FPA was a pioneer of marital therapy (from at least as early as the 1940s) and in training doctors to deal with patients' sexual difficulties. Celebrities like Michael Balint were involved with their training programmes. Sex education in general was also a concern, and became an even higher priority once the main work of birth control provision was taken over by the NHS in 1974.

FPA literature demonstrates the Association's commitment to outreach. Besides producing leaflets in numerous languages for communities for whom English was not the first language, it undertook a number of initiatives to get birth control to groups which needed it but were not using it – for example, by setting up a domiciliary service whereby trained doctors would visit women in their homes.

There was a good deal of controversy during the 1940s and 1950s over the issue of seeing women before their marriage in order to give them advice and fit them with contraceptives, and many precautions were taken to ensure that the women in question were *bona fide* brides-to-be and that the devices would not be used for premarital sex. It was not until the 1970s that the FPA changed its policies in order to provide contraception to unmarried women for whom a wedding was not an imminent prospect. Much earlier however, in 1958, Marie Stopes had left her flagship clinic in central London to the Eugenics Society (in order to keep it out of the hands of the FPA). But since the Eugenics Society was not experienced in running clinics, it drew upon the expertise of the FPA, who realised that this clinic was not bound by the rules of the FPA. As a result, a number of doctors associated with the FPA were able to set up a pioneering clinic for unmarried women (documented in the papers of the Eugenics Society).

With this relaxation of rules about marital status and the final incorporation of birth control provision into the NHS, the FPA increased its efforts in the field of sex education and public awareness of birth control. Particular attention was paid to young people and the desirability of taking precautions: for example, the innovative use of a comic style of presentation in 'Too Great a Risk'.

While the main locus of the FPA's activities was the UK, it also had strong international ties. Health professionals from many countries visited UK clinics for training purposes. There is relatively little material on its relations with the Birth Control International Information Centre, set up in the 1930s in London to coordinate international efforts, but there are several boxes of files on the International Planned Parenthood Federation established after the Second World War, material on the increasing concern with population growth worldwide, and the setting up of Population Countdown in the 1970s. Additional information on international initiatives can be found among the papers of C. P. Blacker and in the Eileen Palmer collection of birth control material.[5]

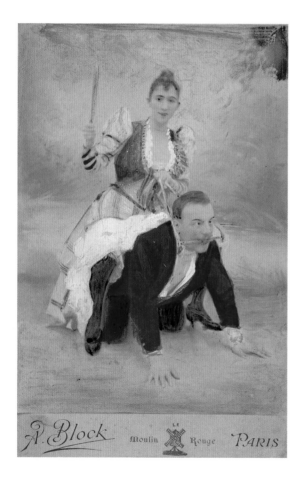

1880s erotica, from the Krafft-Ebing collection of papers

SEX RELATED COLLECTIONS
Krafft-Ebing and Parkes Weber

A range of other diverse issues in sexuality is represented among the collections in Archives and Manuscripts, from the problem of sexually transmitted diseases, to sex education, the pioneering work of Professor Richard von Krafft-Ebing on homosexuality and fetishism,[6] and the activities of the Wellcome Historical Medical Museum in collecting items of erotica.[7] The wide-ranging and fascinating papers of Dr Frederick Parkes Weber (1863–1962) include bundles of correspondence, notes and diverse other material on rare sexual disorders and sexual development, as well as marriage, hermaphroditism and homosexuality between the 1890s and the 1950s.[8]

Marriage guidance and sex education

In addition to the Marie Stopes and Eugenics Society material discussed above, there are a number of other collections of papers of individuals and organisations active in the birth control, sex education and marriage guidance movements. The British Social Hygiene Council was established in 1914 as the National Council for Combating Venereal Diseases, but between the wars took on a much broader remit in pioneering sex education.[9] Edward Fyfe Griffith (1895–1988) was British editor of the journal *Marriage Hygiene* and was involved in setting up the Marriage Guidance Council.[10]

NEWS FROM THE PAST

by Wendy Moore

The staid corners and corridors of a library are not the obvious place for a blinding career revelation. Yet without a doubt it was a first visit to the Wellcome Library which set me on a path that led inexorably to a change in career.

From that first morning when I climbed the marble staircase of the library building at 183 Euston Road – a jaded medical journalist on a rare excursion into historical research – I was enthralled. The names of the medical history 'heroes' carved into the frieze which encircled the main room – Galen, Avicenna, Malpighi, Hunter – meant nothing. The titles on the spines of the volumes stacked from floor to ceiling could have been in another language (and many were). Yet here, away from my usual daily diet of hospital closures, waiting lists and professional rivalries, I discovered a fabulous new world of hospital closures, waiting lists and much, much more – all tinged with the novelty of the past.

My appetite whetted, I soon preferred reading about Claudius Galen cutting the spinal cords of pigs in Roman market places to deciphering more government pronouncements on market forces. Rather than hear of advances in keyhole surgery, I thrilled to the flamboyance of Sally Mapp, so celebrated for her eighteenth-century bone-setting skills that she rode to consultations in a coach and six.

Before long I had enrolled on the Diploma in the History of Medicine course, run by the Society of Apothecaries but based in the Wellcome Library, so that I could devote my Saturday mornings to more historic news. Eventually, I took the plunge and gave up journalism to spend my days in one alcove or another of the Wellcome Library, hoping to add my own volume – a biography of John Hunter – to the thousands already on the shelves.

Working in any library is essentially a solitary and silent venture. Yet every day brought revelations which cried out to be shared – especially with the irrepressible John Hunter as my invisible companion, as bouncy and excitable as a puppy. Every library user knows the experience of suppressing a yell of euphoria at reading the document which slots a long-hidden piece of the jigsaw into place. Equally we have all had to stifle the groan of disappointment when a manuscript reveals we have been led up a blind alley.

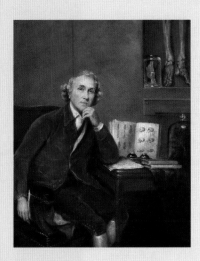

The eighteenth-century surgeon and anatomist John Hunter. Oil painting after Sir Joshua Reynolds

Life with Hunter produced the whole gamut of emotions requiring concealment or disguise. It is not easy to keep down lunch when reading his descriptions of tasting bodily fluids in the corpses he dissected, or to hold back a gasp at his directions for pulling healthy front teeth from children lined up as 'donors' for his transplant experiments. It is hard to stem a chuckle at Hunter's wickedly insightful annotation in a biography of his elder brother William, that 'whatever he was really attached to he was in the strictest sense a miser', or his frank reply to a pupil who accused him of changing his views: 'Very likely I did. I hope I grow wiser every year.'

Most moving of all were the startling life-size engravings of unborn babies within their mothers' wombs in William Hunter's *Anatomy of the Human Gravid Uterus* of 1774. The illustrations, originally sketched by Jan van Rymsdyk, depicting many dissections performed by John Hunter, portray in life-like detail the curling hair and clenched fingers of children who would never take a breath. And in one extraordinary drawing, van Rymsdyk had faithfully reproduced in the membrane covering the baby's spine the reflection of the Georgian nine-paned window by which Hunter had conducted his knifework.

With revelations such as these in store, each time I climb the stairs to the Wellcome Library, I know I will never regret the career switch inspired by that first visit.

❖

of the Sanatorium, New-road; Fell. of Roy. Med. Chir. Soc. and Member of the Council.

HOBBS, John, 35, Southampton-row, Russell-square — Surgeon; Qualification, M.R.C.S.E. Jan. 1, 1819; F.R.C.S.E. 1844.

HOBSON, Nicholas Geo., 5, Great Marylebone-street—General Practitioner; Qualification, L.A.C. 31st Dec. 1834.

HOCKEN, Edward Octavius, 13, Bloomsbury-square—Physician; Qualification, M.D.; M.R.C.S.E. 23rd July, 1841; Physician to the Blenheim-street Infirmary and Free Dispensary; Fellow of the Roy. Med. Chir. Soc.; Corresponding Member of the Med. Society of the Grand Duchy of Baden; Hon. Member of the Abernethian Society of St. Bartholomew's Hospital; Member of the Provincial Med. and Surgical Association, &c.; Author of—1. " A Practical Treatise on Ophthalmic Medicine," part 1; 2. " A Treatise on Amaurosis and Amaurotic Affections, with the Connected Diseases," &c.; 3. " An Exposition of the Pathology of Hysteria, elucidated by a Reference to the Origin, Diagnosis, Symtomatology, Pathology, and Treatment of Hysterical Amaurosis;" 4. " An Essay on the Comparative Value of the Preparations of Mercury and Iodine in the Treatment of Syphilis;" 5. " Observations on Rheumatic Endocarditis and Pericarditis, especially on their early Diagnosis and Treatment."

HOCKLEY, William, 7, Winckworth-place, City-road—General Practitioner; Qualification, M.R.C.S.E. April 1, 1814.

HODDING, Wm Henry, 67, Gloucester-place, Portman-sq.—General Practitioner; Qualification, M.R.C.S.E. May 5, 1826; L.A.C. March 2, 1826.

HODGES, Thomas, 104, Guilford-street, Russell-square —Surgeon; Qualification, M.R.C.S.E.; Jan. 17, 1812.

HODGES, Richard, 17, Upper Barnsbury-street, Islington—General Practitioner; Qualification, M.R.C.S.E. Jan. 17, 1812.

HODGKIN, Thos. 9, Brook-street, Grosvenor-square—Physcian; Qualification, M.D.; Mem. Roy. Coll. Phys. Lond.; formerly Lecturer on the Principles and Practice of Medicine at St. Thomas's Hopital Medical School, Author of a Work on the Pathology of Mucous and Serous Membranes.

HODGSON, Joseph, 1, Norton Folgate — General Practitioner; Qualification, M.R.C.S.E. May 7, 1824; L.A.C. May 10, 1823.

HOGG, Charles, 14, Finsbury-place, South, Finsbury-square — General Practitioner; Qualification, M.R.C.S.E. May 27, 1836, L.A.C. Dec. 10, 1835; contributed to the " Lancet" in 1843 "A case of Varicose Veins," and in 1844 a Paper on " Ovarian Dropsy," &c.

HOGG, John, 71, Gower-street, Bedford-square — General Practitioner; Qualification, M.D. ——

HOLDEN, Luther, 1, Old Jewry—Surgeon; Qualification, M.R.C.S.E. Jan. 19, 1838.

HOLDING, Charles, 13, New Bridge-street, Blackfriars —Surgeon; Qualification, M.R.

14
HUNT THE ANCESTOR: GENEALOGY AND MEDICAL RECORDS

The village of Audlem lies at the southern edge of Cheshire. Dominating the square, below the mediaeval church on its mound, is a nineteenth-century cast-iron monument to Richard Baker Bellyse (1809–77), who practised medicine in the village for forty years. The plinth quotes *Cymbeline*: 'By medicine life may be prolonged, yet death will seize the doctor too.' Medical men and women assist at life's crises: birth, death and much of what lies between. The records they generate can be of great value to the family historian. But they may themselves be the subject of genealogical research. The library's printed and manuscript holdings provide information for family historians looking both for medical personnel and for patients; here is a sample of the sources.

The library's run of the *Medical Directory* is the place where one begins the search for a doctor active at any time from the mid-nineteenth century onwards. The *Directory* tracks doctors' medical lives, recording qualifications, positions held and important publications; it records their eventual retirement and finally death, the latter either through an obituary or by the name simply vanishing silently from the lists. Doctors' places of residence are shown, so successive volumes will reveal their movements from one place to another.

Some entries are lengthy and take up half a column, whilst others are far terser. In some cases this is down to temperament. For instance, the 1845 entry for the eminent pathologist Thomas Hodgkin is a model of brevity and self-effacement, in which his description of what we now call Hodgkin's Disease is mentioned only as 'Author of a Work on the Pathology of Mucous and Serous Membranes'. (By the time of his death twenty years later it has not grown much.) By contrast, next to him the far less well-known Edward Octavius Hocken lists numerous articles under their full titles, and is at pains to make sure that the world knows he is a Corresponding Member of the Medical Society of the Grand Duchy of Baden.

In most cases, however, medical eminence – and the doctor's own priorities – are reflected directly in the length or brevity of the individual's entry as well as in its content. Richard Baker Bellyse's entry is virtually unchanging. In 1817 he passes the examinations to become a Member of the Royal College of Surgeons and Licentiate of the Society of Apothecaries, the two basic qualifications for the nineteenth-century general practitioner. (The *Directory* does, of course, list other qualifications in other doctors' entries, with London's Royal College of Physicians and the various Colleges in Glasgow, Edinburgh and Dublin awarding certificates. Contemporary readers of the *Directory* would have been able to deduce the doctor's precise status – and his price – from the combination of initials after his name. Bellyse's set of certificates is a standard one for a provincial practitioner.) He practises in Audlem for the remainder of his career, adding only the position of District Medical Officer and Vaccinator for the Nantwich Poor Law Union (Nantwich being the local town).

In the fullness of time, an adjacent entry appears for Edwin Swinfen Bellyse, who qualifies similarly but 28 years later and practises seven miles away in Nantwich: almost certainly R. B. Bellyse's son.

Previous page:
A 'model of brevity
and self-effacement':
the distinguished physician
and pathologist Thomas
Hodgkin's entry in the 1845
London Medical Directory

Nineteenth-century
cast-iron monument
to Dr Richard Baker
Bellyse in the Cheshire
village of Audlem

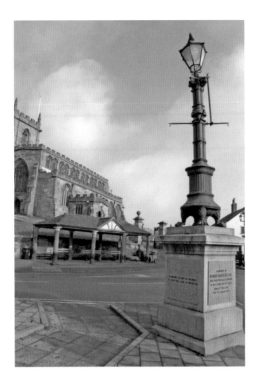

Through its content, but also, between the lines, through its repetitions and absences, the *Directory* paints a picture of a country practitioner as pillar of his community, immersed in his locality and its concerns rather than in the wider world of medicine.

Diaries and account books

The documents produced by local medical practitioners like Bellyse, anchored as they are in a community, are a valuable resource for the family historian. Diaries and account books record visits to patients and treatments, their radius usually the distance one could travel out and back on horseback in a day. The library has an account book dating from the late eighteenth and early nineteenth century, produced by a practitioner in Towcester (Northants) – probably Timothy Watkins, whose family practised medicine in Towcester for several generations.[1] On one side of the book, notes of money received document his work as a man-midwife: 'Lenham's wife, ten shillings and sixpence. Emma Chambers, one guinea. Mrs. Lewis, ten shillings and sixpence …' Litchborough parish is charged two guineas, perhaps for attendance on the poor. On the facing page are outgoing expenses: 'a flannel waistcoat, three shillings and sixpence. Writing papers, twopence. Horse tax, ten shillings and sixpence. Becky and Tommy [presumably servants], eleven shillings and sixpence …' The minutiae of a life are gathered up into this small battered volume. Also present are details of patients seen. The family historian working on the period before civil registration of births, marriages and deaths may have only an individual's date of baptism from the parish records: a record such as this, when it survives, will give the date that the doctor actually attended on the mother and so fill in the missing detail.

Pages relating to childbirths from the account book of a late eighteenth- and early nineteenth-century medical practitioner in Towcester, Northants

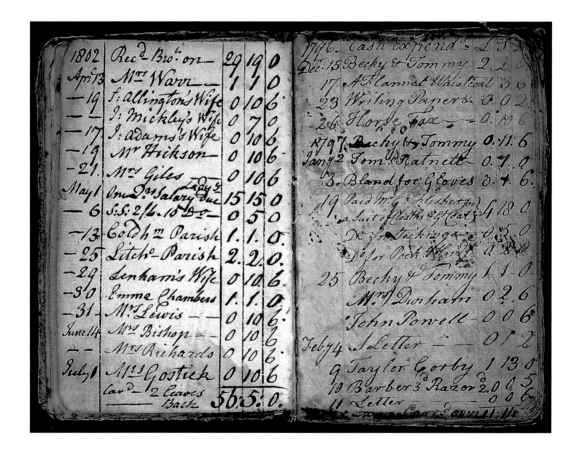

Nursing records

The library's holdings are not confined to doctors, of course. Nurses are also represented and one document captures the birth of the modern nursing profession in a single snapshot. Amongst the thousands of letters from Florence Nightingale in the collection is

List of nurses employed by Florence Nightingale during the Crimean War, 1855

one to Sir John Henry Lefroy, a senior artillery officer who had supported her work during the Crimean War, in which she lists the nurses who served with her at Scutari and Balaclava.[2] It is not necessarily a proud moment for people who may discover an ancestor in this select band, however, since Nightingale spells out bluntly the reasons why some went home, or were sent:

'Invalided'
'Dead'
'Urgent business at home'
'Private reasons'; and, below that, 'Accompanied the above'
'Unfitness'
'Impropriety of conduct'
'Buying and selling for patients in hospital'
'Went home with patient'
'Intoxication'

Before our very eyes Sarah Gamp is getting her marching orders from the nursing profession.

This, of course, is a random, informal snapshot of one small group. In the wake of Nightingale's work various bodies were set up to train nurses, which generated more structured records in larger quantities. The Queen's Nursing Institute was one such body and specialised in the training of district nurses. Its large archive is a goldmine for the family historian.[3] On a basic level it gives the outline of a nurse's career, the date on which she qualified, where she worked and the date of her retirement from the profession, but even more revealingly each nurse was inspected regularly and the assessor's reports, sometimes unsparing, fill the Institute's registers:

'An excellent nurse, careful & thorough.'
'A good average district nurse, rather old-fashioned.'
'A reliable midwife but methods lack finish, brusque in manner.'
'A very good surgical nurse. Thoroughly capable & somewhat outspoken. Manages colliery district well.'
'An average worker. Did not prove amenable in the Home.'
'Very anxious to do well, makes the Home comfortable, but lacks organising powers.'
'Off duty owing to stroke. Died.'

Holloway Sanatorium, Egham, Surrey, founded by the Victorian patent pill manufacturer, Thomas Holloway

Our ancestors stripped bare

So far we have encountered patients only as the list of names in the Towcester practitioner's account book. Runs of clinical records, in which patients move to centre stage, occur at various points in the library's archive holdings, one example being the archives of various private mental hospitals. These vary in extent from the huge archive of the Ticehurst House hospital in Sussex – virtually intact from the late eighteenth century onwards – to stray volumes from institutions such as Camberwell House asylum in South London.

In the middle as regards size is a run of registers from the Holloway Sanatorium in Egham, Surrey, an institution founded – along with Royal Holloway College – by Thomas Holloway on the profits of his patent pill business. Many of the Sanatorium's records appear to have been lost in the 1980s, when a major fire was followed shortly by the Sanatorium's closure. However, those in the library shine a vivid light on the patients there in the late nineteenth and early

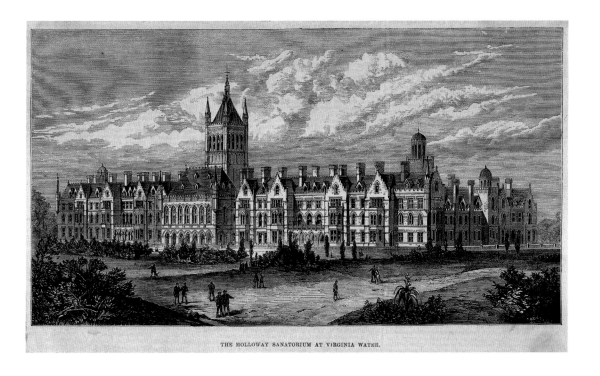

THE HOLLOWAY SANATORIUM AT VIRGINIA WATER.

Condition on Admission—   A. Physical

P. is a dark complexioned girl of Italian(?) type with short curly dark hair — Fairly developed ... is stout — Palate not arched but somewhat asymmetrical — Slight scoliosis. Tongue fairly clean — She presents no P.S. of disease in thoracic or abdominal viscera — Reflexes all very brisk — cranial reflex present — Eyes dark — pupils equal, react very readily to L., A., consensually & to skin stimulation.

She presents no "hysterogenic zones", & there is no ovarian tenderness but she is very "ticklish"—

Catamenia stated to be regular, painless, somewhat profuse ... began at ...

Urine ... 1025. ... turbid with ... urates, urea = 2% ... blood ...

B. Mental   Adolescent Mania.

P. is very variable — usually violent & languid — at times has attacks of screaming & hysterical crying & laughter — is then usually excited & often kicks or hits out impulsively at anyone near her. She shows great animosity towards her parents, especially her mother — & owns to a great lack of self-control, stating that she cannot prevent ...

Opposite and below:
Extracts from Holloway
case notes of the 1890s,
with photographs of
female patients

twentieth century – made still more vivid by the presence of photographs.[4] The stiffness of most Victorian portraits is absent from these photos, the subjects by and large being too wrapped up in their own concerns to pose. They gaze out from the page tense and distracted, cheeky and defiant, rapt by something in the middle distance, lost in dementia, ingratiating, screaming with fury. Beside the photos, there are medical staff reports of their state on admission and their progress, or lack of it: she is 'somewhat less eccentric'; he is 'cheerful, interested, weak-minded' and continues to express a sexual interest in teenage boys; she 'masturbates freely and without shame'; she is worried that people are blaming her for starting the Boer War. Here are our ancestors stripped bare.

In most cases the library's holdings for the family historian do not drill so deeply into personal matters. But as these examples show, they do not simply document medicine as an abstract science: the human scale is never far away. Whether in the conventional framework of a medical career outlined in the *Directory*, leading in the end to a respected burial as 'a man … to all the country dear' (as Richard Baker Bellyse's memorial records), or in the cool assessment of a nursing inspector – 'A good average district nurse, rather old-fashioned' – or again in the confusion and unhappiness of a Holloway patient, doctors, nurses and patients are vividly present as individuals.

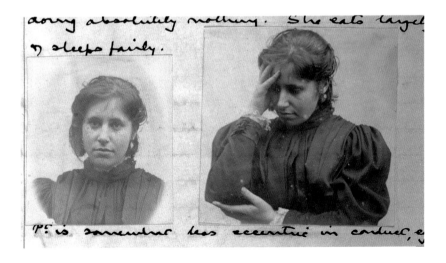

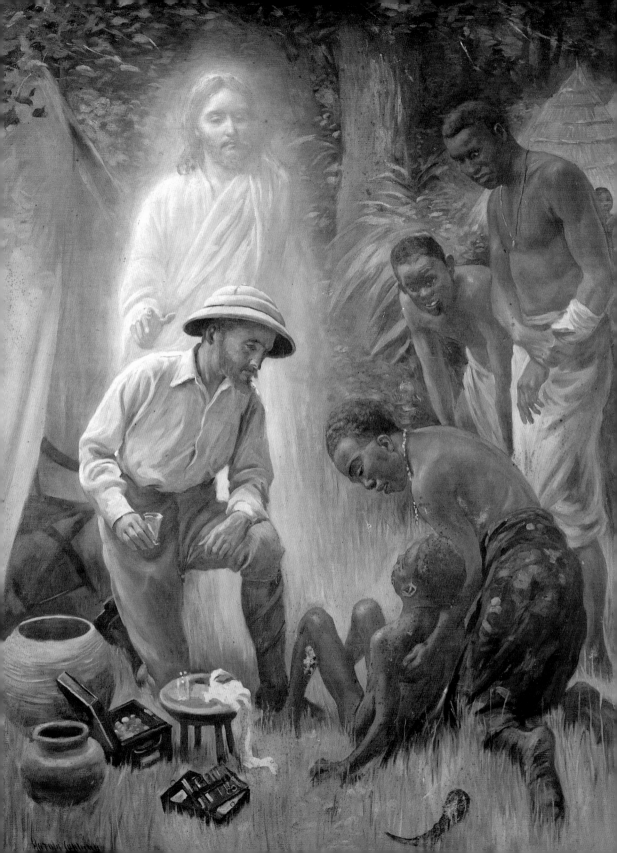

15
HEAT, DUST
AND DISEASE:
TROPICAL MEDICINE,
MISSIONARIES
AND LEPROSY

The term 'tropical disease' is a misleading one. It began to be used at the turn of the last century to cover diseases encountered in imperial medical practice but largely ignored in mainstream European medical education – hence the foundation of a number of Schools of Tropical Medicine, starting with London and Liverpool in 1899. In 1904 Henry Wellcome set up the Wellcome Research Laboratories at Khartoum in the Sudan, and the Wellcome Library contains a wealth of material relating to this and all other aspects of tropical and colonial medicine. This chapter focuses on perhaps the most contentious of all so-called tropical diseases – leprosy.

Leprosy was unknown in the Middle East in Old Testament times, though until recently at least attitudes towards it were rooted in the Book of Leviticus as much as in the teachings of Christ in the New Testament, by which time it may have found its way into Palestine. Victims of the disease are also victims of mistranslation: Old Testament leprosy is not what we call leprosy, but psoriasis, or vitiligo. And while leprosy is generally categorised as a tropical disease, like several others it has less to do with climate than with poverty, malnutrition and insanitary conditions: in the nineteenth century it was rife not only in tropical India but also in near-Arctic Norway, where serious scientific study of the disease began. Yet missionaries in predominantly tropical countries made the disease their own and, in an alliance with colonial medical authorities, revived (or reinvented) the mediaeval notion of it as a spiritual affliction requiring isolation and consolation – not to mention conversion – rather than a mycobacterial disease in need of a cure.

The papers of three leprosy specialists housed in the Wellcome collections reflect the attitudes and dilemmas of doctors with regard to this disease in three different eras.

Henry Vandyke Carter (1831–97)

Two bound volumes of journals kept by Carter between 1848, when he went as a student to St George's Hospital, London, and 1859, after he had joined the Indian Medical Service (IMS) and gone to Bombay, form the centrepiece of the collection.[1] They come to an abrupt end with a fraught account of the rash, possibly invalid and certainly short-lived marriage he contracted there. In sum, they and the family letters that passed between him and his mother and

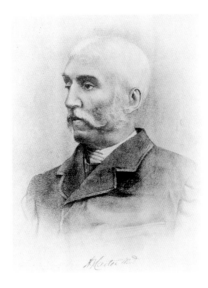

Previous page:
A medical missionary attending to a sick African. Oil painting by Harold Copping, 1930

Left:
Portrait of H. V. Carter

his sister reveal a rather lonely and introverted young man, full of spiritual yearning but racked by religious doubt. The son of a Yorkshire artist, his earliest claim to fame was as illustrator of the original Gray's *Anatomy* (1858).

In relation to leprosy the papers contain a prospectus for an asylum Carter proposed to set up in 1875 for about 150 'pauper lepers' of Bombay. This followed a year's study leave spent mainly in Norway, where he met the 'father of leprology', Daniel Cornelius Danielssen, and his son-in-law Gerhard Armauer Hansen, the discoverer of *M. leprae*, the microbe responsible for the disease (later given the alternative name of Hansen's Disease in his honour). Though personally close, Danielssen and Hansen were on opposite sides in the great nineteenth-century debate over whether leprosy was a hereditary or a contagious disease. Hansen's celebrated discovery might be thought to have put the matter beyond dispute, but it would be some time before leprosy was generally recognised as infectious – if 'the least infectious of all infectious diseases'.

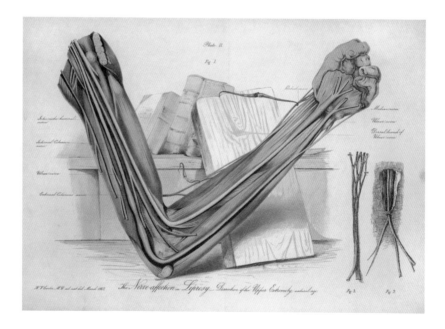

Carter's illustration of nerve damage in the dissected arm of a leprosy victim, 1862

Carter was an early convert to contagionism and did much to spread the word in his books, *On Leprosy and Elephantiasis* and *Report on Leprosy and Leper-Asylums in Norway: with References to India*, both published in 1874 and available in the library. But he was frustrated in his attempts to persuade the government of India to adopt the Norwegian policy of compulsory segregation; apart from anything else it would be too expensive and, in the words of the viceroy Lord Dufferin, 'one might as readily undertake to rid India of its snakes as of its leprosy'.

There are a few letters from concerned activists like the Revd H. P. Wright who, following the widely publicised death from the disease of the Belgian Catholic missionary Father Damien at the leprosy settlement on the Hawaiian island of Molokai in 1889, produced an alarmist publication entitled *Leprosy: an Imperial Danger* that drew heavily on Carter's published work. But by that time Carter had retired from the IMS and, though he remarried and had a second family in the 1890s, was already gravely ill with tuberculosis.

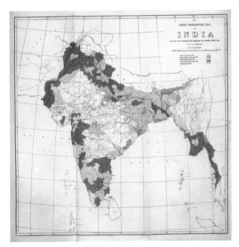

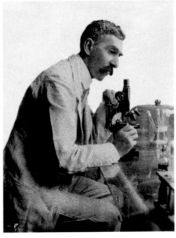

Far left:
Map of India showing the distribution of leprosy, 1890–91

Left:
Sir Leonard Rogers at work

Sir Leonard Rogers (1868–1962)

Leonard Rogers was, according to his friend Ronald Ross, a 'perfect tiger for hard work', and his voluminous papers – diaries, experimental notebooks, drafts of books and articles, as well as correspondence with medical greats such as Ross, Patrick Manson, Robert Koch and William Osler, to name but a few – reflect his many scientific and administrative interests.[2] Like Carter before him, he was an officer in the IMS and he worked on several other diseases, notably kala azar, before he turned to leprosy, just as he was instrumental in setting up the Calcutta School of Tropical Medicine before he co-founded (with Revd Frank Oldrieve of the Mission to Lepers) the British Empire Leprosy Relief Association (BELRA), an organisation – now called LEPRA – devoted to tackling the problems of leprosy scientifically.

Like Carter too, he underwent a conversion – in his case, over the management of leprosy. Until the early 1920s he had supported compulsory segregation, particularly as practised by the Americans in the Philippines, where no expense had been spared in setting up a model leprosarium – a colony within a colony – on the island of Culion. But once he had developed an injectable form of hydnocarpus oil, based on the indigenous Indian remedy of chaulmoogra (and marketed cheaply by Burroughs Wellcome & Co. under the brand name 'Alepol'), he was faced with a dilemma:

> The improved treatment was only of material value in comparatively early cases of leprosy. The only method of control of the disease in general operation was compulsory segregation. Under that system early cases suitable for treatment were all hidden for fear of imprisonment for life. Nothing less than a complete revolution in our 2,000-year-old conceptions regarding the control of leprosy was therefore required …

His papers show how tirelessly Rogers campaigned to phase out traditional leprosaria and replace them with local clinics offering early treatment with Alepol. They also reveal the opposition he encountered from South Africa's Minister of Public Health, Dr J. A. Mitchell, who reacted angrily to having his country criticised for failing to move with the times. In the course of an acrimonious correspondence Mitchell argued – not unreasonably – that Rogers was promising more than he could deliver and was therefore guilty of disappointing leprosy patients, whose hopes had been raised only to be cruelly dashed again.

Rogers lived long enough to witness the real revolution that came in the 1940s with the application of sulphone drugs to leprosy. Only then did it become genuinely possible to speak of a cure.

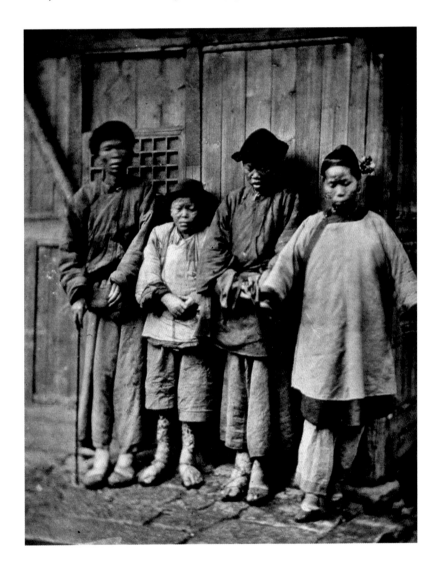

Four people with leprosy photographed outside a wooden hut in Foochow, south-east China – possibly by the photographic pioneer John Thomson, who was there in the late nineteenth century. Henry Wellcome acquired almost 700 glass negatives of Thomson's photographs of mainly Asian subjects in 1921, the year Thomson died, and this invaluable photographic record is housed in the Wellcome Library

*It might be of use to you to know, Sir,
something of the conditions which obtain from
our point of view: segregation without definite
treatment; no system towards a cure; improper
housing accommodation; impure water
facilities; more or less meagre food; dreary
monotony of existence; inadequate hospital
arrangements; severe punishment in specially
made cells (in which solitary confinement
in a cold dark room, or cell, predominates).*

*No wonder the only proper salutation
to the Hon'ble Surgeon General is: Hail, Sir,
we who are put here to die, salute thee.*

*Hoping that it will please you, Sir, to do
all in your power to help us out of our present
state of leprosy.*

A letter to Sir Leonard Rogers from three inmates of the Chacachacare settlement
in Trinidad, 29 June 1924

Stanley George Browne (1907–86)

Stanley Browne went to the Belgian Congo as a medical missionary
in 1936. As a child of poor parents in south London, his imagination
fired by stories of African exploration and missionary activity in the
'Dark Continent', he was already going out to work when he won a
scholarship to study medicine at King's College Hospital, London,
which gave him the opportunity to realise his ambition. He spent three
decades in Africa, mainly at the Baptist Missionary Society hospital at
Yakusu on the banks of the upper Congo, and latterly as Director of
the Leprosy Research Unit at Uzuakoli in Nigeria, where he did
pioneering research on the anti-leprosy drug B663, or clofazimine.

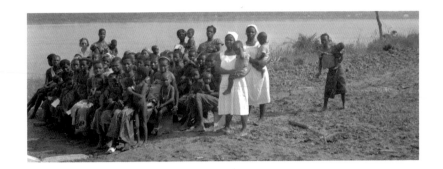

A baby clinic at Yakusu on the banks of the Upper Congo, 1952 – from the papers of the missionary doctor, Stanley Browne

Copious written and photographic material on Browne's time in the Congo – now including a continuous run of letters to his family (up to 1954) – is complemented by documentation of his fourteen years in charge of the Leprosy Study Centre in London (which closed in 1980) and of his frequent travels in later years as an international leprosy consultant.[3]

The papers show how Browne and his missionary colleagues, who had struggled to hold on to the leprosy patients who came to the settlement they opened at Yalisombo, across the river from Yakusu, were on the brink of admitting defeat when the sulphone revolution finally reached central Africa. Word then got around that *Bonganga* (the white doctor) had a new medicine that cured leprosy, and the people who had been deserting Yalisombo in droves returned, bringing so many others with them that demand constantly threatened to outstrip supply. In a vast district with an extremely high incidence of the disease, Browne's achievement was to train and organise a network of *infirmiers*, or medical auxiliaries, 'to embark on a campaign of war against leprosy'.

On a lighter note, there is an account by his wife Marion ('Mali') of how Browne found himself acting as Fred Zinnemann's 'assistant producer' on *The Nun's Story* when the director and cast of the film, including Audrey Hepburn and Peggy Ashcroft, rolled into Yalisombo in their 'huge, gleaming American cars' and delighted the patients – whom they soon learned *not* to call 'lepers' – by involving them in the action.

Though first and foremost a missionary, Browne also preached the secular gospel of *prevention* – prevention of leprosy and, failing that, prevention of disability (and the concomitant stigma) through early recognition and treatment of the disease.

TROPICAL MEDICINE RELATED COLLECTIONS
Sir James Cantlie (1851–1926)

Dr Cantlie was a friend and colleague of the 'father of tropical medicine' Patrick Manson and worked with him in Hong Kong. They were both involved in setting up a College of Medicine for Chinese, and Cantlie became well known for his good nature, his energy and his 'fads'. Like the man himself, his report on *Leprosy in Hong Kong* (1890) is a combination of sound common sense and wackiness – as exemplified in his extraordinary notion that 'house infection' was the cause of the disease, based on Leviticus ch. 14. He became President of the Royal Society of Tropical Medicine and Hygiene and was co-founder and co-editor of the *Journal of Tropical Medicine and Hygiene*.

Cantlie's papers reveal his multifarious interests, which included the physical degeneration of British townsfolk, particularly Londoners (due to a lack of ozone), suitable clothing for boys and girls, first aid and the development of the St John Ambulance Association, military

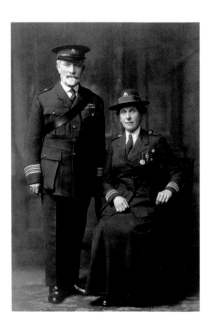

Sir James and Lady Mabel Cantlie in the uniform of St John Ambulance during the First World War

medicine, Robbie Burns and Scottish ballads.[4] His lifelong friendship with the Chinese revolutionary leader Sun Yat-sen is well-documented, including his part in obtaining Sun's release (and thus in saving his life) after he had been kidnapped and imprisoned in the Chinese Legation in London in 1896. Several scrapbook volumes bear witness to his penchant for controversial statements and the largely innocent fun the press had at his expense.

Sir Albert Ruskin Cook (1870–1951)

Albert Cook was enamoured of Africa long before he went there. 'My love grows for my beloved continent every day,' he wrote to his mother from Trinity College, Cambridge, in 1890. 'I am now reading breakfast and lunch *Mackay of Uganda*…' Six years later he set out for that very country with eleven other Church Missionary Society (CMS) missionaries, including Miss Katharine Timpson, a nurse whom he would marry in 1900.

This was the heroic age of both missionaries and imperialism in Africa, and Cook's letters and journals reflect the hardships and excitements of those pioneering days of guns and bibles: Cook even entitled an article he wrote, 'Bullets I have met'. His evangelism might be old-fashioned, but his commitment to building a modern hospital for Africans (in the teeth of considerable opposition within the CMS) was both visionary and impressive, as Henry Wellcome recognised when he footed the bill for Mengo Hospital's new 'Wellcome' dispensary, which opened in 1905 and was said to be 'the best building in Uganda for its size'.

This is mainly a religious war, the heathens v. the Christians. The King hates the Europeans because they stopped his gross immorality, the Chiefs hate us because a Christian is expected only to have one wife & because no slaves are to be allowed, & the people hate us because they say they are obliged to carry loads & to make roads (measures adapted by the government for the good of the country) & because the old heathen customs are dying away.

A letter to his mother from Albert Cook, Namiremba, Uganda, 12 July 1897, during the Nubian uprising

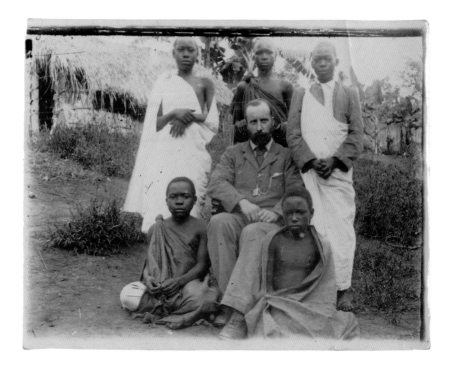

The missionary doctor Sir Albert Cook with a group of African boys at Mengo Hospital, Uganda, in 1897

So it is fitting that Cook's voluminous papers, which include the correspondence and diaries of his remarkable mother, Harriet Bickersteth Cook, as well as material relating to his younger brother Jack who also spent many years as a medical missionary in Uganda and was, along with Albert, the first to diagnose sleeping sickness in East Africa, should be held in the Wellcome Library.[5]

Cicely Delphine Williams (1893–1992)

Dr Cicely Williams was a scion of Jamaica's 'brutal and licentious plantocracy'. But there must have been something in the genes to have produced so outstanding a doctor and humanitarian. In the Gold Coast (Ghana) in the 1930s she discovered a protein deficiency disease she called by the local name *kwashiorkor* (meaning 'the disease of the deposed baby when the next one is born') and had to contend with the supercilious dismissiveness of the overwhelmingly male medical establishment that chose to believe she had misdiagnosed pellagra.

During the last week everything became more and more harassing and disintegrated. When I drove about, the town was full of evacuating and deserting soldiers — most of them Australians — looking utterly disorganised and defeated. They had mostly thrown off their equipment — they were looting the shops or sitting in rows with their boots off down near the quays. They were pushing women and children out of the way to get behind the building when bombs were falling nearby — they were crowding women and children off the boats that were getting away. Many, many of them must have been killed by the Nips in the islands off Singapore. It was a terrible show.

From Cicely Williams, 'Fall of Malaya', undated manuscript

An altercation with the (male) doctor who was her senior led to her transfer to Singapore, where in 1942 she was interned by the Japanese at Changi gaol, an experience of cruelty, hardship and deprivation she later summarised, in a résumé of her personal life, in a single sentence: 'During the war I was interned and had some excellent first as well as second-hand experience of malnutrition.' Nutrition was her speciality and after the war, at an age when many would be contemplating their retirement, Williams started what amounted to a second career as a lecturer and international authority on maternal and child health care. Her crusade was for breastfeeding and she was justly proud of the record of the women's camp at Changi: 'Twenty babies born, twenty babies breastfed, twenty babies survived. You can't do better than that.'

Her collected papers fill many boxes and reflect a life lived to the full.[6] There is much of specialist medical interest, but for the general reader the notebooks and other writings about her time in Changi reveal the essential woman: unselfish, a born leader, always thinking of others, and brave beyond belief.

In Sunday School a teacher was explaining that God made flowers & birds. 'And concrete?' demanded one of the children. 'And aeroplanes?'

From Cicely Williams's Changi notebooks, 1943–45

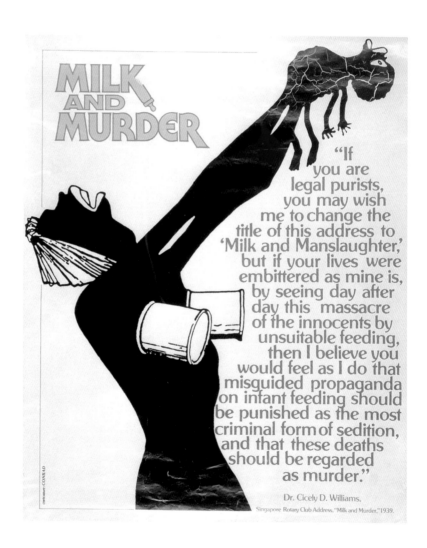

In praise of breastfeeding: a 'Milk and Murder' poster, featuring an extract from Dr Cicely Williams's powerful address to the Singapore Rotary Club in 1939

Acknowledgements

My thanks go, first and foremost, to Julia Sheppard, Head of Research and Special Collections at the Wellcome Library, for inviting me to do this book. The end-product is probably a bit different from what either of us envisaged when we set out (inspired by the excellent *Poets and Polymaths* from the University of Sussex about its special collections). But the journey, though bumpy at times, was always exhilarating. Thanks, too, to Frances Norton, Head of the Wellcome Library, for her hospitality, encouragement and support of the project, and to the Wellcome Trust for making it all possible.

I owe an enormous debt to all the archivists and librarians who, in addition to the daily demands of their jobs, cheerfully took on the task of writing one or more chapters under pressure of short deadlines and then had to put up with further demands from an exigent editor. So a special thank-you to Richard Aspin, Alice Ford-Smith, Lesley Hall, Christopher Hilton, Douglas Knock, Ross MacFarlane, William Schupbach, Nikolaj Serikoff, Julianne Simpson and, once again, Julia Sheppard. Many more members of the Wellcome staff helped in other ways: in particular, Phoebe Harkins, who was so much more than a 'Girl Friday', and Venita Paul, Senior Picture Researcher in the Photographic Library, who gave unstinting support and help with images for the book.

The external contributors were also asked to produce copy at short notice and responded magnificently. My thanks, then, to Sarah Bakewell, Anne Hardy (an inside outsider, rather than an external contributor perhaps), Philip Hoare, Kathryn Hughes, Armand Leroi, Wendy Moore, Robert Olby, Ruth Richardson and Gillian Tindall, for their enthusiasm and professionalism.

I am especially grateful to Sebastian Faulks for responding so gamely to my request for a foreword when I cornered him in the library (my spies having alerted me to his presence there).

A further word of thanks is due to my friend Chris Culpin who, when I started out on this book, gave me the benefit of his own research in the collections, incorporating educational material into the Wellcome Library website. And a special thank-you to Paul Forty, acting for Profile Books, for so calmly and meticulously masterminding the publication process of this book.

My debt to my wife Jenny is incalculable. She is responsible for so much more than the chapter for which she is credited. She was my co-researcher, my most astute critic and my physical as well as moral mainstay. She regularly put together and took apart the wheelchair I had to use in the library and pushed me up the considerable slopes of the underground passage linking the Wellcome buildings on either side of the Euston Road – a task, she would say, she was happy to do so long as I bought her lunch at our destination, the Wellcome's excellent canteen across the road from the library's temporary home.

Tony Gould

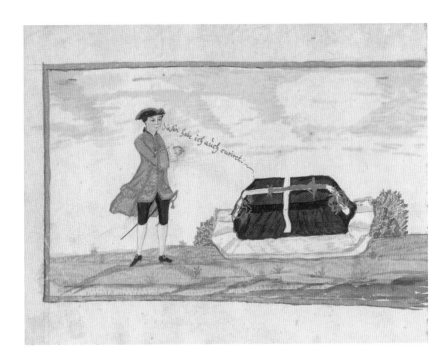

In this mid-eighteenth century German watercolour by Christian G. Gross, a physician, pointing to the coffin of a deceased patient, says 'Diesen habe ich auch curiret' ('I cured him too')

TEXT REFERENCES
Wellcome Library catalogue references for cited texts

Introduction
1 MS.4244   2 RAMC/349

Chapter 1: Collecting the Everyday
1 WA/HSW   3 WA/HMM/CO/Ear/560   5 3418i
2 WA/HSW/ME   4 WA/HMM/RP/Jst

Chapter 2: Repositories of Domestic Knowledge
1 MS.46   6 MS.160   11 MS.3777
2 MS.1026   7 MS.1340   12 MS.7976
3 MS.213   8 MS.1990   13 MS.3712
4 MS.184a   9 MS.363   14 MS.6956
5 MS.761-762   10 MS.7113

Chapter 3: Breakthroughs and Bust-ups
1 GC/48   2 PP/EBC   3 PP/CRI

The Roving Intellect of Francis Crick
1 PP/CRI   2 PP/CRI/D/1/2/1

Chapter 4: A Card Written in Arabic
1 WellcomeIslCal no. 87   2 WA/HMM/CO/HME/37

Chapter 5: Plagues, Pests and Pollution
1 MS.7938/16   4 SA/SMO   7 PP/CED
2 PP/AWD   5 GC/193   8 SA/HVA
3 MSS.6201-6207   6 GC/186   9 SA/PHC

Forceful and Forthright: W. H. Bradley
1 PP/JRH

Chapter 6: Wicked as Ever

1 MSL/B/LON, vol. 1
2 Ibid
3 HIST.G.O/S F.2248
4 MS.7364.69-70
5 MS.8332
6 12566i
7 Rare Books: Ephemera 18
8 MS.7058
9 43542i
10 EPB Bindings: 14
11 Rare Books: Ephemera 18
12 EPB MST.12

Chapter 7: Ministering to Minds Diseased

1 MSS.6245-6790
2 MSS.6220-6221
3 MSS.5157-5163, 8159-8160
4 SA/MAC
5 PP/KLE
6 PP/SHF
7 SA/GAS
8 PP/BOW
9 PP/RKF
10 PP/WWS
11 PP/CPB
12 MS.8166

Chapter 8: By Land and Sea

1 MS.6962
2 MS.7114
3 MS.5875
4 MSS.7679-7680
5 MS.5853
6 MSS.3298-3303,
6182-6200 & 6961-6989
7 Charles Dickens, *Nicholas Nickleby*
(Penguin edition, 1978), p. 350
8 MS.3906
9 MS.5324
10 PP/HAM

Chapter 9: The Elixir of Life

1 EPB Inc. 2.a.24
2 EPB 1114/D
3 EPB 3842/D
4 MS.693
5 MS.239
6 EPB 49072/B
7 MS.524
8 EPB Bindings 7
9 EPB 36700/B

The Many Meanings of Monsters

1 MS.136, Histoires prodigieuses. For a facsimile and translation
(Bamforth, S. (ed.) 2000. Franco Maria Ricci, Milan)
2 43375i, engraving by Taylor, c. 1790
3 Liceti, F. *De monstrorum natura caussis et differintiis*. Padua (1634)
4 Buffon, G. L. L. Comte de (1749–1804). *Histoire naturelle, générale et particulière,*
avec la description du cabinet du roi. De l'Imprimerie Royale, Paris
5 Vrolik, W. *Tabulae ad illustrandum embryogenes in hominis et mammalium, tam naturalem*
quam abnormen. G.M.P. Londonck, Amstelodami (1849)
6 Hirst, B.A. and G.A. Piersol. *Human Monstrosities*. Young J. Pentland,
Edinburgh (1892–1893)
7 Roessler, E. *et al*. 'Mutations in the human sonic hedgehog gene cause holoprosencephaly',
Nature Genetics, 1996, 14: 357–60

Chapter 10: Doctors at War

1 MSS.7034-7035
2 MS.7036
3 MSS.3667-3681
4 MSS.3172, 5316-5318
5 RAMC 95
6 RAMC 630/1
7 RAMC 192-197
8 RAMC 208-212
9 RAMC 251
10 RAMC 2023
11 RAMC 1218
12 RAMC 1816

Chapter 11: A Quick Fix

1 GC 69
2 SA/BOA
3 SA/BMA
4 EPH 494-497
5 MSS.7164-7201

Chapter 13: Wives, Lovers and Mothers

1 SA/FPA
2 PP/MCS
3 SA/EUG
4 PP/CPB
5 PP/EPR
6 PP/KEB
7 WA/HMM
8 PP/FPW
9 SA/BSH
10 PP/EFG

Chapter 14: Hunt the Ancestor

1 MS.6883
2 MS.5479/1/2
3 SA/QNI
4 MSS.5157-5163, 8159-8160

Chapter 15: Heat, Dust, and Disease

1 MSS.5815-5821
2 PP/ROG
3 PP/SGB
4 MSS.7923-7940
5 PP/COO
6 PP/CDW

ILLUSTRATION REFERENCES

Copyright in all illustrations is held by the Wellcome Library, London, except where otherwise indicated below

Key to Wellcome Library holdings

A&M   Archives and Manuscripts
Asian   Asian Collections
CMC   Clinical Medicine Collections
HOM   History of Medicine Collections
IC   Iconographic Collections
MPL   Medical Photo Library (Image Collections)
RB   Rare Books

Front cover

A male *memento mori* figure used for spiritual contemplation, c. 1800, from Wellcome Museum Collection: MPL L0035764

Back cover

A female *memento mori* figure used for spiritual contemplation, c. 1800 from Wellcome Museum Collection: MPL L0035768

Introduction

p. 2: A&M MS.4244
p. 4: A&M MS.4244
p. 6: A&M RAMC 349
p. 7: A&M RAMC 349

Chapter 1: Collecting the Everyday

p. 9: A&M MS.49
p. 10: A&M WF/M/1/PR/F01
p. 13: A&M WA/HSW/PH/E
p. 17 (left): A&M WR 2/30/115
p. 17 (right): IC 13193i
p. 20: IC 14431i (copyright courtesy of the Earl of Harrowby)
p. 22: A&M WA/HMM/RP/Jst/B/2
p. 23: HOM *Handbook to Wellcome Historical Medical Museum* (London, 1920)

Chapter 2: Repositories of Domestic Knowledge

Mr Beeton's Secret

Chapter 3: Breakthroughs and Bust-ups

The Roving Intellect of Francis Crick

Chapter 4: A Card Written in Arabic

Chapter 5: Plagues, Pests and Pollution

Forceful and Forthright
p. 83: MPL L0002227

Chapter 6: Wicked as Ever
p. 84: IC 43542i
p. 87: RB *London's dreadful visitation: or a collection of all the Bills of Mortality for this present year …* (London, 1665)
p. 90: IC 12566i
p. 91: IC 561778i
p. 92: A&M MS.7058/7
p. 93: A&M MS.7058/1
p. 95: RB Ephemera 17

A Serpentine Tale
p. 97: RB E. May, *A most certaine and true relation of a strange monster or serpent …* (London, 1639)

Chapter 7: Ministering to Minds Diseased
p. 98: A&M PP/BOW/L.2/8
p. 101 (left): IC 35111i
p. 101 (right): IC 38621i
p. 102: A&M MS.6783
p. 103: A&M MS.6393
p. 104: A&M MS.5157
p. 108: A&M PP/KLE/A.47
p. 109: A&M PP/KLE
p. 110: A&M PP/WWS/F.7/3

Chapter 8: By Land and Sea
p. 112: A&M MS.5875
p. 114: A&M MS.6962
p. 117: A&M MS.6962
p. 120 (top): A&M MS.5875
p. 120 (bottom): A&M MS.5875
p. 122 (left): A&M PP/HAM/A.31/3
p. 122 (right): A&M PP/HAM/A.31/1
p. 123: A&M PP/HAM/A.17

Young Doctors in Post-Revolutionary Paris
p. 125: MPL M0004481

Chapter 9: The Elixir of Life

The Many Meanings of Monsters

Chapter 10: Doctors at War

The Memory of a Military Hospital

Chapter 11: A Quick Fix

Chapter 12: Goigs and Thankas

Making Honey

p. 171: RB John Villette, *The annals of Newgate; or malefactors register* (London, 1776)

Chapter 13: Wives, Lovers and Mothers

p. 172: A&M PP/MCS/C.51
p. 174: MPL L0029683 (reproduced courtesy of H. Stopes-Roe)
p. 175: A&M PP/MCS/C.45
p. 176: A&M SA/FPA/A.16/9 (copyright Family Planning Association)
p. 178: A&M SA/FPA/A.7/129 (reproduced with permission; copyright SSL International)
p. 180: A&M SA/FPA/A.3/13 (copyright Family Planning Association)
p. 182: A&M PP/KEB/E

News from the Past

p. 185: IC 45666i

Chapter 14: Hunt the Ancestor

p. 186: MPL L0013818
p. 189: photograph, 2007, by Howard W. Hilton
p. 190: A&M MS. 6883
p. 191: A&M MS.5479/1/2
p. 193: IC 23018i
p. 194: A&M MS.5159
p. 195: A&M MS.5159

Chapter 15: Heat, Dust and Disease

p. 196: IC 535948i
p. 198: MPL M0012973
p. 199: CMC H. V. Carter, *On Leprosy and elephantiasis* (London, 1874)
p. 200 (left): CMC *Leprosy in India: Report of the Leprosy Commission in India, 1870–91* (Calcutta, 1892)
p. 200 (right): MPL M0003304
p. 202: IC 35193i
p. 204: A&M WTI/SGB/K.3/1/1
p. 205: IC 561601i
p. 206: A&M PP/COO/K.14
p. 209: A&M PP/CDW/M.52

Acknowledgements

p. 211: IC 583061i

LINKS AND FURTHER INFORMATION

Chapter 1: Collecting the Everyday

The Wellcome Museum for the History of Medicine, comprising those artefacts that survived the culls of the collections as well as newly acquired material, is on permanent display at the National Museum of Science and Industry in Cromwell Road, London. A selection of the most bizarre and interesting can be seen in the 'Medicine Man Two' exhibition at Wellcome Collection, 183 Euston Road, London.

Chapter 2: Repositories of Domestic Knowledge

Manuscript recipe books and associated correspondence and papers are often found within family and estate collections in local record offices.

There are significant accumulations in large research libraries, such as the British Library and the Folger Shakespeare Library.

One or two of the individual manuscript recipe books in the Wellcome Library are very closely related to papers in other collections: Anne Dacre's book is one of several recipe books associated with her held variously in Arundel Castle, Worthing Museum and the Folger Library; Ann Fanshawe's book is a companion volume to her memoir of her husband (British Library Add. MS.41161).

Chapter 3: Breakthroughs and Bust-ups

Fleming's papers are held by the British Library; St Mary's Hospital Alexander Fleming Museum has archives and equipment and one can see the exact spot where Fleming made his discovery.

Florey's papers are now in the Noel Butlin Archives Centre, Canberra, Australia; Countway Library of Medicine, Harvard University, USA holds his lectures for 1965; Nuffield College Library, Oxford University, holds his correspondence with Lord Cherwell; the Woodson Research Center, Rice University, Texas, USA, holds his correspondence with Sir Julian Huxley.

Maurice Wilkins's papers are at King's College, London.

The papers of Brenda Maddox, Rosalind Franklin's biographer, are scattered in various collections including King's College, London; Churchill College, Cambridge; and the Venter Institute, USA.

Watson's papers are at Cold Spring Harbor, USA.

Chapter 5: Plagues, Pests and Pollution

Sir George Newman's diaries are in the National Archives, and other Newman family papers are in the Hereford and Worcester Record Office.

The Imperial War Museum holds papers of Dr Letitia Fairfield concerned mainly with her service in both World Wars and related topics; and some files relating to her work as a Medical Officer for the London County Council may be found among the Public Health Department records now in the London Metropolitan Archives. Some additional material relating to Dr Fairfield is in the extensive archives of the Medical Women's Federation (SA/MWF).

Additional material relating to Dame Janet Vaughan can be found at the Wellcome in the archives of the Strangeways Research Laboratory (SA/SRL), the papers of Dame Honor Fell (PP/HBF) and among the papers of Sir Weldon Dalrymple-Champneys (GC/139). There are several other collections of her papers outside the Wellcome: in the Countway Library at Harvard University; at Somerville College, Oxford; in the archives of the Nuffield Foundation; in the records of the Goodenough Committee (Interdepartmental Committee for Medical Education); and in the Ministry of Health records in the National Archives.

Chapter 6: Wicked as Ever

The proceedings of the Old Bailey – http://www.oldbaileyonline.org/

Chapter 7: Ministering to Minds Diseased

The Wellcome has collaborated with The National Archives to produce and maintain an online database of hospital records and their current whereabouts, Hosprec: http://www.nationalarchives.gov.uk/hospitalrecords/: this includes information on the records of several hundred hospitals which dealt with psychiatric patients at some stage of their existence, held in numerous repositories (mainly local record offices) throughout the UK.

The National Archives at Kew is a major source for the history of psychiatry. Not only does it hold the records of the Commissioners in Lunacy, but also Chancery records relating to cases of alleged lunacy and control over property of lunatics. Records of institutional care are to be found in many local record offices.

Some additional Camberwell House material is held at the Royal College of Psychiatrists, and the great bulk of the records of the Holloway Sanatorium is at Surrey Records Centre, Woking. The Royal College of Psychiatrists retains its own archives and also holds a few items of deposited material.

The British Psychoanalytic Society archives are held at the Institute of Psychoanalysis, along with the papers of a number of leading figures in British psychoanalysis, including Ernest Jones, Freud's disciple and first biographer. Freud's own papers are in the Library of Congress, Washington DC.

Chapter 9: The Elixir of Life

The Young Collection at the University of Strathclyde was donated by James 'Paraffin' Young (1811–83) to support the Young Chair of Technical Chemistry. It contains books and manuscripts on alchemy and early science dating from the fifteenth to the nineteenth century, plus modern support material and reprints. The collection is listed in a printed bibliography, *Bibliotheca Chemica* (2v, 1906), by John Ferguson. (http://www.lib.strath.ac.uk/speccoll/young.htm)

The Duveen Collection at the University of Wisconsin-Madison contains around 3,000 sixteenth- and seventeenth-century works in alchemy and chemistry. It is described by Denis Duveen in his printed bibliography *Bibliotheca Alchemica et Chemica* (London, 1949). (http://www.library.wisc.edu/libraries/SpecialCollections/khunrath/duveen.html)

The Chymistry of Isaac Newton project at the University of Indiana is working to produce a scholarly online edition of Newton's alchemical manuscripts integrated with new research on Newton's 'chymistry'. (http://webapp1.dlib.indiana.edu/newton/)

Chapter 10: Doctors at War

The most important complementary collections in respect of the RAMC Muniments, apart from what is in the National Archives, are in the Imperial War Museum and the National Army Museum.

Chapter 11: A Quick Fix

National Archives at Kew; http://www.nationalarchives.gov.uk/default.htm. Photographs of Sequah and his carriage.

Chapter 13: Wives, Lovers and Mothers

The bulk of Marie Stopes's copious papers are held in the Department of Manuscripts at the British Library.

Chapter 14: Hunt the Ancestor

Wellcome Library biographical and family history resources guide: http://library.wellcome.ac.uk/assets/wtl039833.pdf

Chapter 15: Heat, Dust and Disease

The London School of Hygiene and Tropical Medicine library has much material relating to leprosy, as well as to tropical diseases in general. Also LEPRA and the Leprosy Mission have extensive records of their leprosy-related work.

FURTHER READING

Chapter 1: Collecting the Everyday

Robert Rhodes James: *Henry Wellcome* (Hodder & Stoughton, 1994)

Helen Turner: *Henry Wellcome: The Man, His Collection and His Legacy* (Heinemann, 1980)

John Symons: *Wellcome Institute for the History of Medicine: A Short History* (The Wellcome Trust, 1993)

Ken Arnold & Danielle Olson (eds.): *Medicine Man: The Forgotten Museum of Henry Wellcome* (British Museum Press, 2003)

Chapter 2: Repositories of Domestic Knowledge

Jennifer K. Stine: *Opening closets: the discovery of household medicine in early modern England*, PhD thesis, Stanford University, 1996

Lynette Hunter and Sarah Hutton (eds.): *Women, Science and Medicine* (Alan Sutton, 1997)

Sara Pennell: introduction to *Women and Medicine: Remedy Books, 1533–1865, from the Wellcome Library* (Thomson Gale, microfilm publication 2004)

Chapter 3: Breakthroughs and Bust-ups

R. Macfarlane: *Alexander Fleming, The Man and the Myth* (Hogarth Press, 1984)

R. Macfarlane: *Howard Florey: The Making of a Great Scientist* (Oxford University Press, 1979)

Ronald W. Clark: *The Life of Ernst Chain: Penicillin and Beyond* (Weidenfeld & Nicolson, 1985)

Ronald Hare: *The Birth of Penicillin and the Disarming of Microbes* (Allen & Unwin, 1970)

Brenda Maddox: *Rosalind Franklin: The Dark Lady of DNA* (Harper Collins, 2002)

James Watson: *The Double Helix* (Weidenfeld & Nicolson, 1968)

Matt Ridley: *Francis Crick: Discoverer of the Genetic Code* (Harper Press, 2006)

Chapter 5: Plagues, Pests and Pollution

Michael Warren & Huw Francis (eds.): *Recalling the Medical Officer of Health: Writings by Sidney Chave* (The King's Fund, 1987)

Anne Hardy: *The Epidemic Streets: Infectious Disease and the Rise of Preventive Medicine, 1856–1900* (Oxford University Press, 1993)

Royston Lambert: *Sir John Simon 1816–1904: and English Social Administration* (MacGibbon & Kee, 1963)

Chapter 6: Wicked as Ever

V. A. C. Gatrell: *The Hanging Tree: Execution and the English People, 1770–1868* (Oxford, 1996)

Ruth Richardson: *Death, Dissection and the Destitute* (Phoenix, 2001)

Chapter 7: Ministering to Minds Diseased

Charlotte Mackenzie: *Psychiatry for the Rich: A History of Ticehurst Private Asylum, 1792–1917* (Routledge, 1992)

Eric Rayner: *The Independent Mind in British Psychoanalysis* (Free Association, 1991)

Chapter 9: The Elixir of Life

Ernst Darmstaedter: *Berg-, Probir- und Kunstbüchlein* (Munich, 1926)

Bruce Moran: *Distilling Knowledge: Alchemy, Chemistry, and the Scientific Revolution* (Cambridge, Mass., 2005)

Anthony Grafton & William Newman (eds.): *Secrets of Nature: Astrology and Alchemy in Early Modern Europe* (Cambridge, Mass., 2001)

Chapter 10: Doctors at War

Ian R. Whitehead: *Doctors in the Great War* (Leo Cooper, 1999)

Robert Richardson: *Larrey, Surgeon to Napoleon's Imperial Guard* (revised edn., Quiller Press, 2000)

Mark Harrison: *Medicine and Victory, British Military Medicine in the Second World War* (Oxford University Press, 2004)

Roger Knight: *The Pursuit of Victory: the Life and Achievements of Horatio Nelson* (Allen Lane, 2005)

Chapter 11: A Quick Fix

William Schupbach: 'Sequah: an English "American medicine"-man in 1890', *Medical History*, 29:3, 272–317 (1985)

Roy Porter: *Quacks: Fakers and Charlatans in English Medicine* (Tempus, 2000)

Bill Bynum & Roy Porter (eds.): *Medical Fringe and Medical Orthodoxy, 1750–1850* (Croom Helm, 1987)

William Helfand: *Quack, Quack, Quack: The Sellers of Nostrums in Prints, Posters, Ephemera & Books* (The Grolier Club, 2002)

Mike Saks: *Orthodox and Alternative Medicine: Politics, Professionalization and Health Care* (Continuum, 2003)

Chapter 12: Goigs and Thankas

GOIGS

Amadeu Pons i Serra: 'Quin goig de ... goigs!', *BiD: textos universitaris de biblioteconomia i documentació*, juny 2005, núm. 14, <http://www2.ub.es/bid/consulta_articulos.php?fichero=14pons.htm>

Javier Portús Pérez and Jesusa Vega: *La estampa religiosa en la España del antiguo régimen*, Madrid: Fundación Universitaria Española, 1998

John Marston: 'A month at the Wellcome Institute', *Friends of the Wellcome Institute newsletter*, 1995, no. 8, p. 7

THANKAS

Gyurme Dorje: 'A rare series of Tibetan banners', in N. Allan (ed.), *Pearls of the Orient: Asian Treasures of the Wellcome Library* (London, 2003), pp. 161–177

L. Austine Waddell: *Lhasa and Its Mysteries: With a Record of the Expedition of 1903–1904* (London, 1905)

Marianne Winder: 'Two Tibetan thankas', *Friends of the Wellcome Institute newsletter*, 2000, no. 21, pp. 6–7

Marianne Winder: *Catalogue of Tibetan manuscripts and xylographs, and catalogue of thankas, banners and other paintings and drawings in the Library of the Wellcome Institute for the History of Medicine* (London, 1989)

Chapter 13: Wives, Lovers and Mothers

Audrey Leathard: *The Fight for Family Planning: The Development of Family Planning Services in Britain, 1921–74* (Macmillan, 1980)

June Rose: *Marie Stopes and the Sexual Revolution* (Faber, 1992)

Richard A. Soloway: *Demography and Degeneration: Eugenics and the Declining Birthrate in Twentieth-century Britain* (University of North Carolina Press, 1990)

Chapter 14: Hunt the Ancestor

Wellcome Library biographical and family history resources guide: http://library.wellcome.ac.uk/assets/wt1039833.pdf

Chapter 15: Heat, Dust and Disease

Paul Brand, with Philip Yancey: *Pain: The Gift Nobody Wants* (Marshall Pickering, 1994)

Tony Gould: *Don't Fence Me In: Leprosy in Modern Times* (Bloomsbury, 2005)

Zachary Gussow: *Leprosy, Racism and Public Health: Social Policy in Chronic Disease Control* (Westview Press, Boulder, Colorado, 1989)

ABOUT THE
WELLCOME LIBRARY

Sir Henry Wellcome started collecting books, manuscripts, prints and pictures from his student days, although his first recorded purchase for the library dates from 1897. His agents acquired a vast number of items for his library and museum, but the library was never open in his lifetime. It opened to the public in 1949, at 183 Euston Road, in the building specially designed by Henry Wellcome to house his collections. The library has grown since then and now occupies several floors of the same building, refurbished in 2007 and named Wellcome Collection.

The library's holdings are continually being added to, by purchase, gift and deposit. Following Henry Wellcome's lead, a holistic approach has been adopted in order to acquire resources comprising the record of medicine past and present. The library's holdings thus cover an extraordinary depth and variety of materials and information, making it one of the world's greatest collections on the history of medicine from earliest times to the present day.

In addition to 700,000 printed books, printed journals, and a wide range of electronic journals, there are 70,000 rare books and periodicals published before 1851, 600 incunabula (books printed before 1501), iconographic and picture collections of 100,000 prints, drawings and paintings, plus image and sound collections. Unpublished manuscripts in the Asian collections and in Archives and Manuscripts (which include both papers of individuals and records of organisations) are in over 70 languages, and date from c. 1100 BC (a papyrus prescription) up to the present. Electronic resources include Wellcome Images, with 160,000 photographs and photographic reproductions, a virtual 'Turning the Pages', and 'Uncover' – an interactive, touchscreen-based application which enables visitors to search and explore some of the riches within the library's collections.

The library has a broad appeal, relevant to specialist historical scholars as well as those interested in contemporary biomedicine. Opening hours and further information can be found at http://library.wellcome.ac.uk

Wellcome Collection, 183 Euston Road, London NW1 2BP

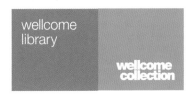

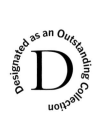